The Diet Struggle

A simple, easy to follow guide to
weight loss and living healthy.

Linny Harris

Table of Contents

Introduction

Do you wake up thinking about what you are going to eat today? How much time do you spend thinking about food, looking forward to your next meal or craving something you know you shouldn't eat? There's the first thing that you need to address, when you think too much about what you are going to eat then you are giving too much power to food.

The average person works 40 plus hours a week and may have children and some sort of personal life that gets squeezed in after work and on weekends. Finding time to prepare healthy meals and go to the gym is not an easy task. The goal here is to provide direction on how to fit exercise into your everyday life and to take another look at food and its purpose. We will also look at popular diets and the mental aspect of dieting.

How many diet books have you already read...but you are still struggling. Many spend a lot of time explaining the science of weight gain and what is fat. They may provide you with a jump-start meal plan that the average person will have a hard time sticking to. And they may give you an exercise regime that you feel you would need to be an athlete with lots of time on your hands to keep up with.

You probably already know the basics, you need to eat more fruits and vegetables, exercise every day, drink lots of water and don't skip breakfast. Knowing what to do and actually doing it is what many struggle with. So we will talk about one the most important aspects of losing weight and keeping it off which is the mental aspect of it.

I'm not going to sugarcoat the truth (we want to avoid sugar literally and figuratively); it's time you stop looking for a quick fix diet or special pill to take and accept that losing weight takes work and a lifetime commitment. You have to be ready to change the way you eat, the way you think about food and ready to incorporate exercise into your life...are you ready to do that? Only then will you be able to stop the diet struggle.

Before we begin, let's throw in just a little science and math; if you want to get an idea of where you are at currently and determine where you want to be here is the formula to determine your BMI (Body Mass Index):

BMI (Body Mass Index) = multiply your weight in pounds ____lbs. x 703 then, divide this number twice by your height in inches. If you're overweight your BMI will be 25 to 29.9 and if you're obese, you're BMI is 30 or greater.

Another statistic to look at is your Waist Circumference, if your waistline is over 31.5 inches for females and over 37 inches for males that is considered overweight. Waist circumference over 35 inches in females and 40 inches in males significantly increases the risks for heart disease, diabetes and impaired ability to perform activities of daily living.

Some common reasons so many are struggling with their weight include:

Super-size syndrome = excessive sized meal proportions as seen with all you can eat buffets or places we don't even get out of the car to consume.

The ill motive psychological affect utilized in advertising that promotes unhealthy foods and dietary lifestyles.

The hidden empty calories found in the additives of sugar and other carbohydrates get the public addicted to craving for specific food products that contribute to obesity and disease over time.

The American lifestyle of lazy, convenience, unbalanced, fast food restaurants and packaged foods.

Studies show that watching four or more hours of TV a day doubles your risk of diabetes and obesity.

Because having a healthy lifestyle has been important to me over the years I have researched and studied books, articles, etc. on weight loss and fitness and want to share that knowledge with you. I also enjoy cooking and creating meals that are healthy, delicious and fun to make so I have included some food "quickies" for breakfast, lunch and dinner and some delicious recipes for when you have more time to cook. I'm not a doctor so it is a good idea to consult one before making any major changes to your diet and exercise regime especially if there is concern about supplements you may start taking.

The intention of this book is to encourage you to live a healthy life by providing a direct and simple guide with straightforward advice plus easy meals and recipes. It's an easy read with advice and tips you can utilize every day, then in six months you can read it again to remind you of those good things you were doing for about four months.

I also want to encourage you to find passions in life other than food, find the joy and happiness eating healthy and getting exercise can bring you. Make yourself a priority each and every day; reward yourself with a massage or facial...things other than food that feel great and provide a benefit to your overall health. If you are dealing with stress find other ways to relieve it besides food; more and more successful people are using meditation to relieve stress and improve their focus. It's something I do daily and find it very beneficial for both my health and career.

Alright now, it's time to take control and stop struggling...so let's get started.

Chapter One: Preparation

Prepare the Mind

To lose weight and keep it off you have to work on your mental attitude. You have got to stop looking at changing the way you eat in a negative way or you will always struggle. You have got to stop looking for quick fixes. You have got to get down to your subconscious in the way you think of food, eating and exercise.

I'm not talking about telling yourself you like eating salads when subconsciously you are thinking I want a pizza. But you've got to clear your mind from the negative thoughts of eating healthy and find healthy foods that make you happy and you feel good about eating. Stop thinking of it as dieting, it's not dieting; it's about living and eating healthy and you will find that this lifestyle feels great!

This is what you need to ask yourself before eating; will I feel good about eating this? Let's take bread for instance, you have a choice between sourdough bread and wheat bread...the wheat bread is good but the sourdough is better so you want the sourdough bread. But ask yourself, will I feel good about eating it? Or you can eat the wheat bread, which still tastes good but when you think about how good it makes you feel to make the healthier choice it will actually taste better than the sourdough. By thinking of how good eating certain foods will make you feel it will make them taste better and you will enjoy eating them. Don't listen to people who say that reduced fat mayonnaise doesn't taste as good as real mayonnaise...some people have a mental attitude that just because it's healthy it doesn't taste as good. Let go of that mental block and realize that healthy food does taste good and the fact that you feel good eating it makes it taste so much better!

My point is I'm not going to lie to you and say that a slice of thin crust veggie pizza tastes better than a slice of pepperoni and sausage pizza; but I'm going to choose the thin crust veggie pizza because it is good, it will satisfy my desire for a slice of pizza and I will feel good about eating it and making the better choice. When you combine all that then it does taste better than the pepperoni and sausage slice.

This will be the turning point for you, when you finally accept that the short temporary satisfaction of certain foods is not worth it; that you can enjoy making good decisions and taking control of what you eat instead of letting food control you. Living a healthy, active life is so much better than that hamburger. I enjoy when I go grocery shopping and when I get to the checkout line I am proud of what I have in my cart.

Something most people who are slim and fit have in common is they are happy eaters. They don't obsess over food and are happy with the healthy choices they make. You have to have a positive relationship with food and keep it in perspective. They eat to live, not live to eat. Think of food as just food, it is fuel for your body that you can also enjoy. Food is not the enemy, your body needs food and cutting back too much will do more harm than good.

There are times when I think I would really love to have some pizza and wonder if I should call Domino's tonight? Then I tell myself I will splurge next weekend on a pizza and most the time when next weekend comes around I no longer have that craving. It's alright to splurge a little sometimes in order to keep yourself from losing control altogether but limit it to only occasionally and keep it in small portions. You can use that if you need to as motivation to stay on track for two weeks then you can enjoy something special. But again be careful with this that you are not giving too much power to the food by using it as a reward.

Another obstacle many face in losing weight is the people we live with. Your spouse or children don't need to lose weight and they want the white bread and the pepperoni pizza so what do you do? They don't mean to be an obstacle but you have not confronted them with the facts or informed them of how you feel and what you need. Talk to them and tell them how you feel, what losing weight means to you and how this isn't just about the way you look but your health. Being overweight leads to so many health issues so this is your life we are talking about. They love you so of course they will want to support you in losing weight and improving your health but you need to make them aware of this.

Even if your family members do nott need to lose weight eating healthier can only enhance their life and you need to point that out. There are other health issues that eating certain foods can lead to such as high blood pressure, high cholesterol and diabetes. Eating foods high in saturated fats can lead to high blood pressure and heart disease. Eating foods high in sugar or simple carbs can eventually train your body to be less efficient at processing blood sugar and lead to diabetes. So even if those around you do not need to lose weight they can only benefit by eating healthier and making better choices with food. We would all be better off if we stopped focusing on the temporary enjoyment from the taste of food and more on the purpose of food and the long-term effects.

And if you have children teach them to eat healthy so hopefully they don't have to face the same struggles you are. Involve the people around you in living a healthier lifestyle and making good choices. Of course there can always be compromises, instead of one large pepperoni pizza get a medium pepperoni and a medium thin crust veggie (or my favorite a thin crust with chicken, spinach and feta cheese). However in the food and recipe section of this book you will find many choices that will definitely please everyone and they won't even realize they are eating healthy!

So remember that you are in control, not the food. Before choosing something to eat ask yourself "will I feel good about eating this?" And if the answer is no then don't eat it. Keep in mind how you will feel after you are done eating…and you will find that when you make these good decisions the feeling you will have is so much better than how that food would have tasted. When making food choices focus on how you will feel about eating it; and think about what your goal is and how you want to look to give you the strength to make the right decisions. Practice mindful eating, being conscious about what you are eating and how much. Listen to your body and stop eating when it tells you to stop, you don't have to clean your plate. And just like with anything else it will get easier with time to make these decisions.

Stress can be a major roadblock to losing weight; being a happy eater helps alleviate some of that. But if you have stress in your life find other ways to relieve it. Make yourself a priority, you need to be a priority and find ways to relax and find enjoyment. When you find yourself stressed out do you stop exercising and turn to food for comfort? You come home from work and order a pizza because you don't feel like cooking or have the energy (stress can zap your energy if you let it). Then you notice how much weight you've gained and stress out more about that; and it can be a vicious circle.

Don't think of food as comfort, there are other ways to deal with stress such as using daily affirmations or write in a journal to express your frustrations. Come up with your own mantra such as "I have the Power" or "Make it Happen" or "I can do this, and I WILL do this", something you can use when you are feeling weak.

Studies have shown meditation is a great stress relief; just a few minutes each day take time to sit and quietly re-center yourself. Quiet your mind and just be still. Focus on the stress leaving your body and think about the positive steps you are going to take each day. There are books and many guides to meditation available to help you get started.

Also when you're heading home stressed and you have no energy don't swing by that fast food joint; there are several recipes and quick food ideas in this book that are quick, easy to prepare but still comfort food. Or you can prepare a nice dinner and use that time cooking as a stress reliever. Exercise is also a great stress reliever and we will discuss that more later.

You have to take control and avoid excuses...it's not easy but you have the power to do this. Start taking control now and hold yourself accountable. Keep your eye on the prize and every day remind yourself what is your motivation; remember why you want to lose weight and how good it will feel when you reach your goal. Think of a positive affirmation for yourself and write it down so you can refer to it and reaffirm the message on a daily basis or as often as you need it. Have you been using food as a crutch or for comfort and if so, write down your feelings about that and how you are going to change it. Then write down how you want to see yourself in six months; not just physically but mentally and emotionally.

So now you understand the need to prepare yourself mentally for changing how you eat, how you think about food and how you want to live your life. What's more important, your health or a hamburger?

The trick is to change your environment and habits so you are setting yourself up for success. Talk to your family, friends or roommates and let them know you are making some life changes to lose weight and improve your health so they can provide support.

Prepare the Kitchen

Clear your kitchen of junk food and stock up on healthy alternatives. Even if you have kids you can provide healthier foods for snacking such grapes, sugar-free Jell-O, apple slices and string cheese. If its chips go for the healthier options such as baked chips so if you are tempted to snack on some chips it's a better option for you but keep it a small amount. Baked tortilla chips and salsa is also a good option or veggies with a natural low-fat dip. Some instant oatmeal that is low in sugar with fruit is also a great snack for you and the kids. And get rid of the soda for both you and the kids; it's ok to drink once in a while but should not be the daily drink of choice. Juice with no sugar added is a better choice for the kids or fruit flavored water.

Stock up on herbs and spices to provide flavor without the fat such as ones mentioned in chapter 3. Other staples for the kitchen are 100% whole wheat bread, brown rice and/or quinoa, whole-grain cereal, beans, mustard, low fat mayonnaise, whole-grain crackers, eggs, skim milk (or almond milk), Greek yogurt, nuts, fresh vegetables and fresh fruit such as apples and blueberries.

Prepare the Body

Cleanses can help to "clean the body" and prepare your body for the change of eating healthier; and you can lose a few pounds quickly with a cleanse but they are not long term solution.

By eliminating caffeine, sugar, alcohol and preservatives for a week or two you can work on eating "cleaner" and reset your body. Eating clean means sticking to whole foods and choosing lean proteins, fresh vegetables and fresh fruit. This is a much healthier option than using one of those cleanses that have you drinking special concoctions, just stick to eating organic, whole grains and vegetables to help flush the waste from your body.

While a weight loss cleanse can help get rid of toxins, it's important to understand the side effects that you may experience. Not all weight loss cleanses are created equal, and if you don't heed the precautions, you may end up in worse shape that you started in. Some side effects include headaches, dizziness, insomnia and loose bowels.

Once the cleanse is over you'll likely feel healthy and happy, better than you have in a long time. This is because the cleanse helps to get rid of toxins that have been building up inside your body. You may also notice that you have tons of energy, much more than you did before.

Sleep is also a key factor for losing weight, those who get more sleep lose weight and those who lose weight sleep better. So make sure you get plenty of sleep each night; 7 – 8 hours per night is recommended.

Chapter 2: Supplements and Popular Diet Plans

Where weight loss pills are concerned such as fat burners and appetite suppressants, its best to avoid them...they tell you to take them with a healthy diet and exercise which is where the weight loss will result from (not the pills) and many have potentially dangerous side effects. Remember there is not a get quick weight loss that will work in the long term, so you can't rely on pills. The best appetite suppressant is water; drink a glass of water before a meal and the water will help fill you up quicker.

There are some vitamins and herbs that have shown to possibly help in weight loss, these include:

Calcium

There have been studies showing people who took a calcium supplement lost 26% more body weight and 38% more body fat than those who ate the same diet but did not take the supplement. Another study showed those who got their calcium from low-fat dairy instead of the supplement lost even more.

When your body doesn't get enough calcium, it triggers fat cells to store fat and get bigger. Additionally, calcium builds strong bones and teeth and aids muscle function.

Cayenne

Thermogenic herbs have shown to help activate the cells in the body and make you burn calories more rapidly. This includes red peppers, which can jump-start your circulation and gets your blood flowing. The substance capsaicin that's found in cayenne helps the body to burn fat.

CLA – Conjugated Linoleic Acid

Research has shown that CLA aids in reducing body fat, building lean muscle mass and boost the resting metabolic rate. CLA is found in beef and full-fat dairy products so since you limit the intake of these foods consider a supplement.

Chromium

Chromium has shown in some studies that it regulates glucose metabolism, which helps control blood sugar levels. It can also help build muscle tissue. You can get chromium in beans, broccoli, eggs and whole grains or as a supplement.

Cinnamon

Another that is reported to aid in lowering blood sugar is cinnamon; it has been shown to help prevent insulin resistance which means it may help slow sugar to pass through your stomach more slowly thus suppressing the blood-sugar spike. Try sprinkling cinnamon on your toast, oatmeal, some apple slices or in your coffee.

Vitamin D

Vitamin D is necessary for adequate insulin secretion; it is also aids in the absorption of calcium for bone strength. Studies have found that people with lower levels of vitamin D are more likely to be obese; especially in menopausal women.

Flaxseed

Flaxseed can help fill you up so that you eat less; it can be taken as a whole seed or ground flaxseed. There is also flaxseed oil that provides essential fatty acids and anticarcinogen which helps strengthen the heart.

Green Tea

Research shows that the substance found in green tea known as catechins can speed up metabolism and helps burn fat. Based on studies aim for 3-4 cups of green tea a day to get the benefits; adding lemon will enhance the benefits. Green tea supplements are also available. *Black tea after a high-carb meal may decrease blood-sugar levels after meals which means you would feel full longer and have fewer food cravings. Researchers credit the polyphenolic compounds in black tea for suppressing rebound hunger.

Selenium

Selenium can be a contributing factor in maintaining a healthy weight by assisting with a healthy thyroid and plays an important role in vital bodily functions. Selenium can be found in seafood, liver, lean red meats, garlic, sunflower seeds and whole grains.

Turmeric

Found in curry powder, turmeric contains curcumin, a yellow pigment that's been shown to combat free radical and inflammatory damage, and could also help protect against memory loss. Try it in your scrambled eggs.

Tyrosine

Enhances mood, increases energy, speeds metabolism. Also may improve memory.

White Kidney Bean

This is used to aid with blocking carbohydrates; it is reported that the extract decreases the calories absorbed from carbohydrates. This doesn't mean you can take some white kidney bean extract then eat some pasta and it will block all those evil carbs; however it could potentially allow you to eat some carbs while losing weight.

Additionally,

Taking a daily multivitamin with minerals has long been considered nutritional "insurance" to cover dietary shortfalls. Choose one based on your age and sex then take daily or when you feel your diet is adequate in providing the daily vitamins your body needs. Although keep in mind it is always better to get your vitamins from food.

Meal Replacements

Using a meal replacement can help control calories and be beneficial, experts say, as long as it's part of a lifestyle that includes exercise and a well-balanced diet. Look for a meal replacement that is low in fat, calories and sugar; look for ones high in protein and fiber to keep you full longer and at least 200 calories (typically if it's under 200 its considered a snack, over 200 calories is considered a meal).

If you have trouble estimating portion sizes, find yourself eating too often or typically choose foods high in fat and calories, meal replacements may work for you. We all know that losing weight is one thing, but keeping that weight off for one, two or even three years or longer is a completely different story. For people who really have trouble changing their eating habits permanently, using one meal replacement per day may be just the ticket to keep weight from coming back. Use meal replacements for no more than 2 meals such as have a shake for breakfast; eat a healthy meal for lunch then another shake for dinner. This will make meal planning and portion control easier. For variety add small amounts of fruits and/or plain non-fat yogurt but keep in mind the calories you are adding. Or if you are using a prepared shake or meal bar such as Slim-Fast or Special K supplement it with some fresh fruit or vegetables on the side.

But just like other diet plans, meal replacements aren't for everybody. If you need the taste of real food and prefer to chew rather than drink your meals, you're probably better off sticking to healthy foods, not meal replacement shakes and bars. A meal of six baby carrots and a turkey sandwich on whole-wheat bread with mustard and dark green lettuce is just as healthy as a 220-calorie meal replacement shake.

Popular Diets

There are a lot of diet plans and programs, some are good and some are a waste of time and money; some can even be dangerous. Don't fall for the false promises that these fad diets offer. We all want to find an easy way to lose weight and lose it quickly but if we listen to our common sense we know that pills or fad diets are not the answer. Remember if it sounds too good to be true, such as "eat what you want, you don't have to exercise, just take this pill and you will lose weight", your common sense should tell you it is too good to be true. You may lose a few pounds on the latest fad diet but it will come back and usually with a few extra pounds.

The reason you are reading this book is you have been struggling with losing weight, you have possibly tried various diets and it keeps coming back. It's time to accept that to lose weight and keep it off means you have to change the way you eat permanently and include exercise in your life. So it's time to accept you have to make a lifestyle change of eating right and making exercise a part of your life. I know I'm repeating myself here but I want to make sure you get it...it's time to start your new life of eating healthy and exercising and it's time to embrace this new life.

There are some diet programs such as Jenny Craig, Nutrisystem and Weight Watchers that are good programs and can help you lose weight if you need some assistance. But keep in mind that you still need to learn how to eat and make your own choices. If you rely only on following the program then once you stop the weight will come back.

Weight Watchers is beneficial for the support you receive, the online service and applications. It is economical and has a proven track record and probably one of the best choices for value and effectiveness.

Nutrisystem is the most affordable meal inclusive plan; they provide the meals and offer a choice in plans in varying lengths of time (14-day, 28-day). Their program focuses on foods with a low glycemic index which controls blood sugar levels leading to weight loss. So there is a balance of good carbs, proteins and fats then you can add fruits and vegetables.

Either way don't just blindly follow the program, use it to help you learn portion control and how/what to eat so you can maintain your weight loss once you are off the program and on your own.

Chapter 3: Helpful Hints

As mentioned in the previous chapter, think about what you are eating and you will actually start enjoying being creative with making meals healthy. I love pasta and when I make it on occasion I will take the standard amount and cut it in half then make up the difference with lean meat and vegetables. For example take a small amount of angel hair pasta; while the pasta is cooking sauté in a large pan some vegetables in olive oil with garlic and basil such as mushrooms, green onion and red peppers. Add some chunks of chicken or for a quick addition add some turkey bacon bits. Then toss the pasta in with the vegetables and last add some feta or goat cheese. There are so many variations; you can sauté asparagus or broccoli and cauliflower which are actually quite good sautéed as opposed to steamed. Use any kind of vegetables you like then add cooked chicken, shrimp or beans for protein. And you have a delicious, healthy meal.

And speaking of chicken, a great time saver is to buy a bag of frozen chicken breasts and cook the entire bag in a crock-pot. In the morning before you head to work or start your day put the frozen chicken with a little seasoning in the crock pot, add a little water, broth, olive or coconut oil so they don't get dry and let it cook all day. Now you have cooked chicken breasts that you can use during the week in salads, in sandwiches or toss in some pasta or with brown rice or quinoa.

Sunday is a great prep day so it's easy to stick to healthy foods during the week when work can limit your time. Boil a carton of eggs so you will have hard-boiled eggs for the week; either for breakfast or to add to salads. You can also make a large bowl of steel-cut oats then during the week scoop out a cup of oatmeal topped with some fruit for breakfast with a hard-boiled egg and you have a fast well-rounded breakfast that will keep you full for hours.

Also take the time to chop up vegetables such as green onion, peppers, cucumbers, etc. to use during the week. If you have a big dinner on Sunday night use the leftovers for Monday night or for lunch; then Tuesday cook some chicken breasts in the crock-pot and have chicken for dinner that night when it's hot and fresh served with vegetables. Then use the remaining cooked chicken during the rest of the week for lunch and/or dinners.

And remember to use spices; spices and herbs add flavor without adding fat and calories. Cinnamon is a great spice in the morning to help keep your blood sugar level. Sprinkle it on your cereal, buttered toast, oatmeal, on apple slices or any fruit, or on your peanut butter and apples. One of my favorite breakfast treats is a whole wheat waffle topped with almond butter sprinkled with cinnamon then topped with a drizzle of sugar free syrup...delicious! An herb I always have around is dried chopped chives; add them to eggs, vegetables, pastas and sauces. When you go to the grocery store stop at the herbs and spices aisle and pick up some new ones you don't have until you have a wide selection at home, then experiment with them on different foods and get creative.

As already stated you need to drink a lot of water; thirst often will feel like hunger causing you to eat more because you feel hungry when actually if you had drank some water that hunger would diminish. Studies have shown those who started each meal with a tall glass of water dropped more weight over 12 weeks and shed it more quickly compared with dieters who skipped the water and just started eating. Your body needs water, start the day with water and drink it before every meal. If you've just eaten and still feel hungry drink some water before eating more and see if your hunger goes away. Another reason to drink some water before going back for more food is it takes 20 minutes you're your brain to get the signal that you are full; so eat slowly then drink some water and most of the time that hunger will go away.

And don't say I don't like water; it has no taste so it's not that you don't like it you just don't enjoy it because it has no taste...so get over it and drink the water! Keep a bottle of water on hand that way I can carry it around, take some in the car and keep one on the nightstand. It's a good idea to drink some water when you first wake up to rehydrate after a good night sleep.

And if you need some flavor try adding slices of lemon or orange to a glass of ice water. You can get the refillable water bottles with a diffuser to add fruit. Or try a splash of cranberry juice to sparkling water and drink it from a martini glass for a special occasion. Be creative but remember not to add too much of anything with sugar.

Another tip you may have heard is to never skip breakfast; if you don't your body goes into starvation mode so your metabolism slows to a crawl to conserve energy. Someone I know who struggles with her weight had told me often she doesn't like to eat breakfast and that she loses more weight when she doesn't eat breakfast; I've heard this several times because she is constantly losing then gaining weight. Then after lunch she would talk about how full she is...maybe she overate because she was so hungry. So listen to the experts and give your body what it needs which is fuel in the morning to start the day. For best results eat breakfast within an hour or so of waking up, even if you're not hungry! Morning time low blood sugar can produce a brain chemical designed to mask hunger pangs which may be why some do not feel hungry in the morning (not me, I wake up hungry). Try to have a breakfast that will keep you full and focused until lunch so it should include protein and fiber. But even if it's just a hard-boiled egg or a piece of whole wheat toast with almond butter just eat something to give your body the fuel it needs in the morning.

Many find it very helpful to keep a food journal and jot down what you eat throughout the day, which will make you more aware of what extra calories are slipping in without you noticing. Studies have shown people who kept a food journal lost twice as much weight as those who didn't. Journaling also gives you insight to your eating habits...do you skip meals or are you eating frequently? And be sure to include what you drink, many forget to include the calories they drink such as the coffee with sugar and cream in the morning, that fruit juice and soda and that wine or cocktail with dinner. The drinks, especially coffee drinks and alcohol can add a lot of calories and sugar to your daily intake. So include EVERYTHING in your food journal that you put in your mouth.

And always, always, always read the labels and know what you are eating. Don't just focus on calories or fat content...some foods will have "low fat" on the package but they increase the amount of sugar to make up for it or "sugar-free" products will have more fat. Read the label and look at the calories, fat, sugar and sodium content. Also look at how many servings this is for; I checked out a bottle of flavored green tea and read the label for the sugar content, it wasn't bad so I purchased the tea then while drinking it I read the label again and realized that it was 2.5 servings in a bottle. So multiplying the amount of calories and sugar by 2.5 made this a worse decision than I thought. Read the label paying special attention to calories, fat, sugar, sodium and number of servings, then compare a few and go with the one that is the best overall.

Of course you won't have to worry about reading labels too often if you are choosing whole foods such as lean meats and fresh fruits and vegetables, they are not packaged...right? Preservatives and additives are not your friend, the fewer the ingredients on the label the better. Later in the book I go over some "power foods" which include dairy, lean meats, fruits and vegetables; these are the things you want to fill most of your cart with.

Here are few more tips:

Drink green tea; research shows that drinking 3 cups of green tea a day reduced body weight by 5 percent in three months. This is due to the antioxidants in green tea that seem to help burn calories and hinder inflammation that leads to obesity.

Avoid processed foods; there is no greater diet destroyer than highly processed foods such as chips and cookies. This is a huge obstacle for dieters now that there are so many "100 Calorie" snacks and processed foods that are marketed as diet foods. Most processed foods are simple carbs that will not fill you up and they also rev up dopamine production making you feel good and wanting to eat more. Any food that has a long expiration date is not something you should put in your body, those preservatives and additives will sabotage the good you put in your body. Stick to whole foods such as fruit and vegetables that are high in fiber and will reduce hunger. And choose natural foods when possible; if you get natural peanut butter and pour the oil off the top you will save about 20 calories and 2 grams of fat plus you are putting less preservatives in your body. It also leads to better skin; toxins make their way out through the skin so the more natural and organic food the better for your skin. The fewer the ingredients the better; and only one ingredient is best!

In addition to drinking water before your meal try starting off with a broth-based soup which will help fill you up before dinner.

Eat slowly; make your goal to be the last one to finish eating. Try putting your fork down between bites. By eating slowly you avoid overeating by giving your brain time to let you know when you are full. And stop before you are too full, once you start feeling stuffed you ate too much.

Choose high-fiber simple carbs; these good carbs raise blood sugar slowly which helps nix cravings and keeps you feeling full. So you will avoid the "white" carbs such as white bread, and white rice. Stick to brown rice and whole wheat. Keep in mind it needs to say "whole" wheat and not just wheat.

Allow some "good for you" fats such as avocados, olive oil and nuts; small amounts of healthy fats satisfy you longer and slow down digestion.

Avoid sugar, especially artificial sweeteners; artificial sweeteners like the kind found in diet soda can confuse your body and trick you into craving more sugar and other foods; they can also lead to internal inflammation and premature aging (sugar also leads to inflammation). So if you think you are doing right by drinking diet coke all day think again; an occasional diet soda is fine but you are not doing your body any favors by drinking it constantly. A good alternative to regular cane sugar is raw coconut sugar, but it's still sugar so keep it in moderation.

Don't overdo cutting back on food and deprive yourself; studies show those who slash their calorie intake too much had higher levels of stress hormones like cortisol and adrenaline which in turn can send your blood sugar soaring. Eat regular meals and snacks but control the portion and eat the right foods.

As previously stated sleep is vital to good health and to healthy weight. Too little sleep may actually work against you and cause you to actually lose muscle mass. Research has shown those who sleep less (6 hours or less) feel hungrier. Aim for 7 to 8 hours of sleep per night.

Diet friendly dishes...splurge on nice dishes and glasses when having dinner, you will find you will slow down and enjoy dinner when it's served in something nice. Also the dinner plates should not be too big; if you have a big plate you will want to fill it up. Stick to smaller plates and bowls.

Points to Remember:

- Dink plenty of water; you can add fresh real lemon or cucumber slices. For best results, drink four 8 ounce glasses (32 ounces) in the morning, then two 8 to 10 oz. glasses of water just before every meal and if you skip a meal you must still drink a your water. Preferably No: sodas, fruit or sugary drink, synthetically sweetened drinks, caffeinated drinks. These all lead to dehydration, acid irritation to digestive track, or adrenal fatigue in the end.
- Get most of your calories from food, not from drinks.
- Eat healthy...try to get mostly vegetables, then proteins, and last carbohydrates for energy and maintaining a healthy weight. Try to eat organic, hormone free, antibiotic free, free range, wild caught, local farm produced foods. Try to eat at least 3 meals a day with healthy snacks in between (fruits and vegetables).
- Avoid refined sugars, salt and processed foods.
- Think before you eat; keep a photo of how you want to look or an outfit you want to fit into hanging on the refrigerator or somewhere in the kitchen. Take a moment to think about if you are truly hungry and about your weight loss goals before you grab something to munch on.
- Keep portions under control; don't eat straight from a box or bag...prepare your portion in a bowl or on a plate then put the rest away. Use

small plates and bowls and break up meals you are saving into individual portions instead of in one large container.

- Eat slowly, put your fork down between bites and enjoy each one. If you are eating with someone enjoy a conversation with them, talking between bites will slow you down even more. Only eat until you are slightly full then stop.
- At work, keep small portions of healthy snacks for mid-morning and/or mid-afternoon. If you want to have protein bars know the calorie count, fat and sugar in each bar so that it is in the snack range (under 150 calories) and not a meal.
- DON'T skip meals, thinking I will skip lunch so I can have a heavy calorie meal for dinner...eat a light lunch and find a way to scale back the calories at dinner.
- When going out to eat or to a party eat a small healthy snack before so you won't be as tempted to over-indulge.
- Exercise, you must get some form of exercise in every day if not twice a day to **increase** your: oxygen intake, lean muscle, metabolic set point, blood flow for growth and development, and decrease your: stress levels, chances of heart attack, healthy exercise should consist of walks (without the cell phone), yoga or stretching, hiking, bike riding, gym, runs, etc.
- In between keep yourself moving every day; walk around your house or clean the house. Turn on music instead of the television, music that makes you want to dance and move around.
- Get plenty of restful sleep, minimum of 6 hours but 7 to 8 hours is preferable.

Chapter 4: Exercise

You hear commercials and see advertisements saying you can lose weight without exercising…if it sounds too good to be true then it probably isn't true. You wonder "how can they promise this if it isn't true" but unfortunately the diet industry isn't regulated very well and they can say just about anything without much recourse.

Exercise is an important part of losing weight and maintaining a healthy weight not to mention it's important for your overall health. So if you are one of those that hate exercise you need to get over it and accept that exercise is a necessary part of a healthy life. We talked about changing your mental attitude towards food and eating; you also need to work on your mental attitude towards exercise.

 Exercise helps you protect against colds and flu; it produces mood-enhancing chemicals like serotonin, dopamine and norepinephrine and eases stress. Not only are you burning calories when you exercise but you increase the calories burned while at rest. You're adding lean muscle, your heart is healthier, you're getting stronger and slimmer…remember this every day when you're debating about exercising. And if that's not enough exercise can slow the aging process and can significantly reduce your cancer risk.

There are lots of excuses for not exercising; the biggest excuse is lack of time. It's ok to ease into an exercise routine by just getting up and moving. When you get home from work you are exhausted and you just want to plop down on the sofa and zone out in front of the television...but when that happens tell yourself to get up.

Get up! Get up! Just start moving while watching the television; you can start off with walking in place and then step it up by doing side to side steps (that's where you step to the right then back to the left) and you can add in a little squat when stepping to the side. Then you can add to it by raising your arms while stepping side to side; hold your hands palms up at your shoulders then when you step to the right raise your left arm like you are pushing something heavy up and again on the other side. Fit in some exercise in the morning by stretching out while you are blow drying your hair then do some "Counter squats" and "Counter push-ups" (described below). Do some squats while brushing your teeth. Find other movements you can do while watching your favorite shows but get up and move for at least 20 minutes instead of just sitting on the couch.

Walking is a great way to start an exercise regime then build up from there. When walking try adding some variations such as walking backwards for a minute or shuffling sideways to challenge your muscles in a new way, work different angles and improve your balance.

Dancing is another way to get you moving and have fun while you are at it, either watching one of those musical singing or dancing shows on TV or turn on some upbeat music and just start dancing. Not only will you feel better and less stressed after a busy day at work but you will sleep better.

If you don't want to go to a gym then try using exercise videos; there are so many out there to choose from at different skill levels. Find something you enjoy that contains both cardio and strength training and from these videos you can pick up some basic moves that you can do anytime and anywhere.

So if time is an issue fit in the 20 minute movement workouts during the week and a bigger longer workout on the weekends. Then work your way up to working out every night; alternating short ones with longer ones. You can also do three or four shorter workouts, 10 minutes, throughout the day...you can do that, right?

Here is a simple plan for a workout schedule:

Monday, Wednesday, Friday and Saturday or Sunday – 20 minute movement workout

Tuesday, Thursday and Saturday or Sunday – 40 minute workout with cardio and strength training (start with 5 minutes of cardio, then weight/strength training, then end with 5 minutes of cardio)

Put your workouts on your calendar like other appointments with a reminder; by having it scheduled in you are more likely to stick to it.

For strength training you don't even need equipment, there are many exercises you can do utilizing your own body weight. But it's a good idea to have some basic equipment at home to use such as 3 and 5 pound weights, a stability ball, or kettle bells. These are inexpensive items that don't take up space and you can do so much with them. If you have the money and space for a treadmill that is great but if not then a stair-step costs very little and can be tucked away under the bed.

Now we have overcome the time objection and there is plenty you can do without leaving the comfort of your home. However if you need more structure and commitment to exercise there are so many gym options, check out the gyms in near your home or work. There are gyms that cater to women and provide a structured work out such as Curves, or gyms that provide more options and classes. If you have a friend to go with it makes it more fun and you can hold each other accountable. Working out at home, at the gym or a combination of both, figure out what works for you and do it keeping in mind this is not temporary but a new way of life for you.

Here are some exercises you can do at home:

Jumping Jacks

This is a great start to get your heart pumping; keep your arms straight as you bring them up to your ears.

Jump Rope

It will be difficult at first, but build up to doing it for 1, 3, 5 then 10 minutes; it works your upper and lower body so it's a great calorie burner.

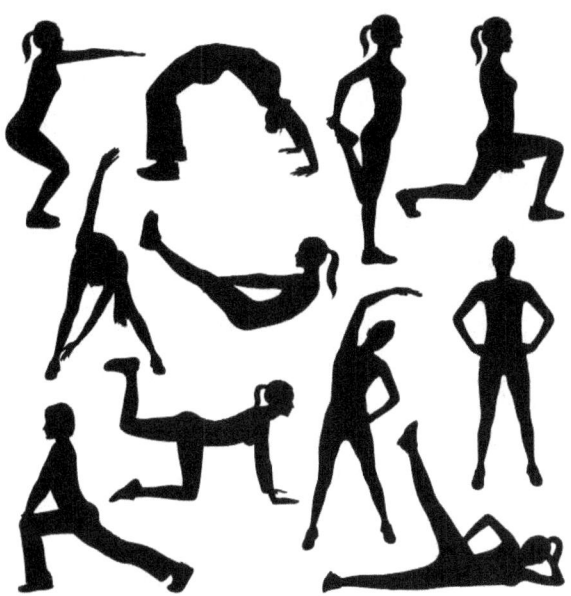

Simulated in-line skating

Stand with your feet hip-width apart, your knees slightly bent; take a big step back and to the side with your left leg behind your right leg then do the same with your right leg back behind your left as if you were skating. Either swing your arms or punch each arm forward as you skate.

Cross Knee Lift

Stand with your feet hip-width apart, hold your arms up bent at the elbows; raise your right leg and bring your left arm down pointing your left elbow to your right knee. Quickly repeat on the other side and rotate back and forth.

Side Leg Lifts

Lie on your side with the leg on the bottom slightly bent and the top leg straight; the bottom arm holding your head and the top arm bracing yourself in front on the floor. Raise the top leg straight up slowly then down and repeat 8-10 times. Repeat on the other side.

Rear Leg Lifts

Kneel on your hands and knees, extend your left leg out behind you bent at the knee and lift 8-10 times pushing your heel towards the ceiling. Repeat with the right leg.

Counter Push Ups

Stand at arm's length in front of your kitchen or bathroom counter, lean forward and place your hands shoulder width apart on the edge of the counter then bending at the elbows push up and down using the counter. This is a great exercise you can fit in while getting ready for work in the bathroom or when finishing up doing the dishes.

Counter Squats

Again using the kitchen or bathroom counter and stand at arm's length away hold the counter as you squat at the knees like you are sitting in a chair then stand back up and repeat 8-10 times. For a little extra when you stand back up raise up on your toes and lower which will work your calf muscles.

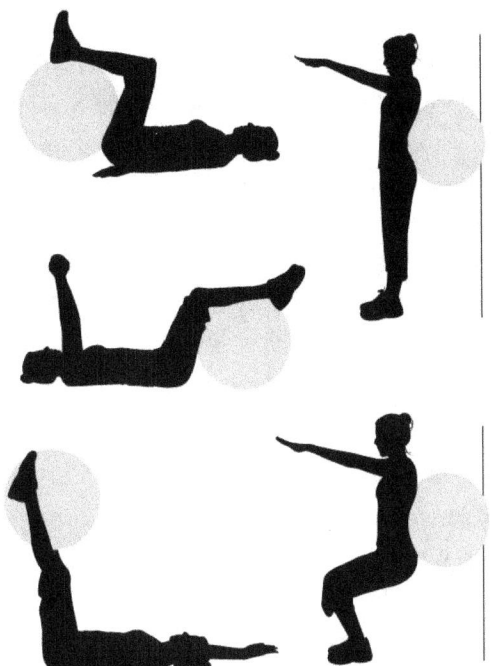

Stability Ball Squats

Using a bare wall stand with the stability ball between you
and the wall at your lower back; leaning back against the
ball lower yourself at the knees while the ball rolls up your
back. For extra strength training do this while holding either
3 or 5 pound dumbbell's in each hand at your side.

Stability Ball Leg Lifts

Lie on your back with your feet on the stability ball and your
hands tucked under your butt; using your feet on the ball
lift your butt off the floor slowly and lower.

Stability Ball Crunches

Lie on your back, legs bent on top of the stability ball; cross arms across your chest and raise your head and shoulders off the floor by pulling up with your stomach muscles (careful not to strain your neck).

For your lower stomach while on your back wrap your legs over the stability ball and while gripping it with your legs lift the ball off the floor using your lower abs.

Stability Ball Curls

Sitting on your stability ball and holding your dumbbells in each hand at your sides curl your arms up to your chest. Additionally work the back of your arms by holding arms up with the dumbbells in each hand, bend elbows so that the dumbbells are behind your ears; slowly lift up towards the ceiling. And another workout for the arms, shoulder and chest is to lie back on the stability ball with your upper back resting on the ball and knees bent keeping your back straight; holding a dumbbell in each hand extend arms out at shoulder level then raise arms toward the ceiling so that the ends of the dumbbells meet in the center.

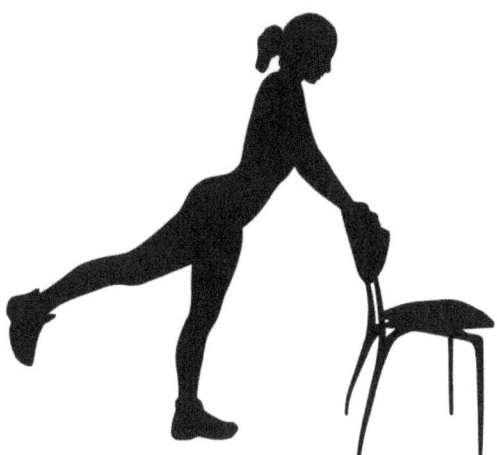

Bar Stool Leg Lifts

Sitting on a barstool or regular chair, place your hands
around the seat of the chair on each side of your legs, with
your legs hanging down lift them as if there is a bar across
the top of your ankles then slowly lower them. Repeat this
and you will feel the muscles working in your thighs.

Bar Stool or Chair Ab Crunches

Sitting with your butt close to edge of the seat, legs at a 90
degree angle, raise your knees up as you feel your stomach
muscles tighten, then lower and repeat.

These are some great exercises you can do at home at any
time. And as a tip, keep your sneakers out to remind you
about working out; in the morning put out your workout
clothes for the day so you have to look at them.

Another form of exercise to consider is yoga; it works the muscles and can also be a tremendous stress reliever. It's a common misconception that you have to be able to do all the poses to even try it. Anyone at any level can do yoga and work your way to the more flexible positions. You can purchase yoga videos to start at home or start taking classes.

Also make sure you move around when you are at work, don't just sit at your desk on your computer all day. Get up and move, walk around the office if possible or climb the stairs if there are some (keep some flats or comfortable shoes at the office to change out of your heels if necessary). If possible get a pedaling machine, one that will fit under your desk that you can use while on the computer. Get up to talk to a co-worker instead of emailing or calling; or at least stand while on the phone.

Even when sitting work your muscles; squeeze your glutes and hold (nobody will know) or lift your feet up on your toes working your calves. Find something in your office that weighs about 3-5 pounds that you can curl or lift over your head and work your arms.

If you travel you can walk the airport during layovers instead of sitting; lift your suitcase or carry it instead of rolling it. Use the above exercises in your hotel room, or use the gym which almost all hotels now have.

When shopping park away from the door so you have to walk a little further; and when grocery shopping make the effort to go put your cart away instead of leaving it by your car in the parking lot (don't be lazy).

Involve your friends and family, get them to take walks with you or for a hike. Plan active events such as bowling or mini-golf. You could also visit a museum or take dance lessons. Get some backyard games to play with the kids or with friends such as Frisbee, badminton or croquet. Go for bike rides when weather permits. Play interactive video games on PlayStation or Wii. Volunteer to help at a shelter or with animals, you get a bonus of doing something good while being active.

So you see there are a multitude of exercises and activities you can start doing now. The only thing holding you back is yourself, just take that first step and move around.

Chapter 5: Power Foods

The right foods can help you drop pounds; a daily multivitamin is helpful but getting the essential nutrients from real food is preferable.

Here is a list of foods that can help you stay full longer, increase your metabolism, curb cravings and lead to a slimmer, healthier you.

Eggs

Eggs have had a bad rap for a long time, they are rich in protein to combat cravings and control hunger. Eggs are also a great source of zinc which can make you feel more awake so it's a great choice for breakfast. And you don't have to skip the yolks altogether, much of the fat and calories are in the yolks but so is most the protein and the vitamin B12 which is needed for fat breakdown. So don't skip all the yolk, use one yolk for every two or three eggs.

Berries

Berries such as blueberries, strawberries and raspberries are loaded with vitamin C and antioxidants; plus they are high in fiber and low in calories. Blueberries also help protect the brain from free-radical damage and provide brain-boosting antioxidants. Toss them in salads, mix them with yogurt, cereal and smoothies.

*Strawberries and salmon share a power food feature, they both boost serotonin levels in the brain much like an antidepressant.

Salmon

The omega-3 fats in salmon are good for the heart and improve insulin sensitivity which helps build muscle and decrease belly fat. And the more muscle you have the more calories your body burns. Opt for wild salmon which has lower levels of PCB contaminants than farmed salmon.

Lentils/Beans

These are high in protein and fiber which helps to stabilize blood sugar levels and keeps you full longer. Beans are also high in iron, magnesium, potassium and zinc...all good things for the body. Try to use fresh beans and cook them instead of canned beans when time permits.

Nuts

Nuts such as almonds are high in protein and in alpha-linoleic acid which can speed up the metabolism of fats. They help build muscle and fight food cravings. But they are also high in fats so eat in moderation. Walnuts are one of the richest dietary sources of serotonin, a chemical in your brain that helps create calm and happiness. So they can also be a "feel good" addition to your diet.

Chicken Breasts

White meat chicken without the skin is a leader for lean protein and a great source for coenzyme Q10 which assists in skin cell turnover. They are easy to prepare in several ways and can be added to just about anything as a protein source.

Tuna

Tuna is also a great source for lean protein; but don't destroy the good by adding fatty mayo, keep it light by using a small amount of low-fat mayo or try mixing it with hot sauce, pepper and some fresh lemon juice. Or just add some tuna to your salad. Tuna has been shown to help lower cholesterol and help your body process fat.

Tofu

For our vegetarians/vegans this is a great source of protein but can also be enjoyed by everyone; it's delicious marinated or tossed in salads and pasta. It also provides amino acids as well as isoflavone which helps muscles recover after exercise.

Tomatoes

They are high in vitamin-C, lycopene and beta-carotene; these can help decrease your risk of cancer and coronary artery disease. They are beneficial with reducing inflammation and some studies show they may help allergy sufferers.

Leafy Greens

These include kale, spinach, arugula, Swiss chard, radicchio and romaine lettuce; these are good sources of fiber, vitamin C & K, folic acid, lutein, and four essential minerals: calcium, magnesium, iron and potassium. Ways to include them are add arugula to your sandwich, layer chard in a healthy lasagna or add spinach to omelets.

Artichokes

This fiber-rich plant contains more bone-building magnesium and potassium than any other vegetable. It's also rich in vitamin C and in antioxidants that can cut the risk of stroke. Ripe ones feel heavy for their size.

Bell Peppers

Bell peppers are low in calorie and fat-free but big in flavor; they are also high in fiber making them a great addition to salads, pasta, pretty much everything. Red peppers are high in antioxidants, vitamin A and C.

Chili Peppers

These stimulate the metabolism; act as a natural blood thinner and help release endorphins to put you in a good mood. They are also rich in vitamin A and help fight inflammation.

Quinoa (pronounced Keen-wa)

This is an amazing food, it can replace pasta, rice, and oatmeal...its nutritional composition is better than most grains. It's a whole grain that is high in protein and fiber to keep you full and satisfied. Alternate it with sweet potatoes and brown rice.

Yogurt

Particularly Non-fat plain Greek yogurt; its strained so even the non-fat versions are thick and creamy. And due to the lack of liquid it means there is more protein than ordinary yogurt. It has the healthy bacteria known as probiotics and is a terrific source of B vitamins, protein and calcium. It's a trifecta of carbs, protein and fat that will stave off hunger and keep blood sugars level. Use yogurt in place of sour cream and mayonnaise.

Oats

Unlike many other carbohydrates, oats digest slowly so they do not have the effect on your blood sugar as other carbs. All oats are healthy but the steel-cut and rolled oats which are minimally processed have more fiber making them a more filling choice. They also provide muscle-friendly energy. Instead of breadcrumbs, add oats to your turkey meatloaf.

Sweet Potatoes

A great vegetable loaded with vitamin C, potassium and fiber which mean no drastic insulin jumps and less fat on your hips. A sweet potato a day also helps protect against Alzheimer's, liver disease, HIV, cancer, heart attack and stroke. Top a baked sweet potato with yogurt and honey and a dash of cinnamon.

Apples

An apple is a great appetite suppressant; eating an apple before a meal can lead you to eat fewer calories. They are high in fiber and the antioxidants in apples can help prevent metabolic syndrome, a condition marked by excess belly fat. The also contain quercetin, an antioxidant that has been shown to act as a natural antihistamine and block substances that cause allergy symptoms.

Prunes

Prunes, or dried plums, can help whittle the waist by causing you to eat less; prunes are high in fiber and its chewy fiber so you eat is slower. Prunes also help to strengthen your bones and boost your energy so they make a great snack.

Dark Chocolate

The flavonoids in dark chocolate fight inflammation and help reduce the risk of heart attack and stroke. Chocolate also has mood-boosting properties. Stick to dark chocolate with at least 70% cacao and due to the high calories limit it to a small amount per day.

Avocado

We all know that avocado is high in fat so moderation is the key, but it's a healthy fat and is filling leading to satiety. Add avocado to sandwiches instead of mayo for the creamy texture.

Olive Oil

Like avocado's, olive oil is a healthy fat that increases satiety curbing your appetite. It also has anti-inflammatory properties; chronic inflammation has been linked to metabolic syndrome.

Here are a few suggestions/recipes to incorporate these super foods into your diet:

Banana-Almond Smoothie – blend one cup skim milk, 1 ½ tbsp. almond butter, 2 tsp. ground flaxseed and one medium banana.

Power Smoothie – blend 1 cup low-fat Greek yogurt, 1 cup blueberries (fresh or frozen), 1 cup carrot juice, and 1 cup fresh baby spinach.

Fruit and Yogurt – 6 ounces of non-fat Greek yogurt, 2 tsp. honey and mix with 1 cup of strawberries or blueberries.

Egg and Mushroom Scramble – in a small amount of olive oil sauté sliced mushrooms, fresh spinach leaves and chopped green onion; stir in lightly beaten eggs/egg whites and scramble.

Oatmeal and Apples – prepare oatmeal (instant or steel-cut), add diced apples, chopped nuts and cinnamon.

Pumpkin Pie Oatmeal – combine 1/3 cup canned pumpkin, 1 cup oatmeal, 1 to 2 tsp. brown sugar and other spices of your choice such as cinnamon, nutmeg, or pumpkin pie spice.

Healthy "Cole Slaw" – mix 1 ½ tbsp. light mayonnaise with 1 tbsp. Greek yogurt, 1 tsp. lemon juice and ¾ tsp. Dijon mustard; toss with store bought package of broccoli slaw. Optional: add sliced almonds and grapes.

Quinoa and Black Beans – heat a can of black beans (as a time-saver) with about a cup of sliced mushrooms, ½ cup of chopped red onion and 1½ cups fresh spinach; simmer about 3 minutes. Serve over cooked quinoa.

Quinoa Salad – cook quinoa according to directions and let cool. Then in a large bowl, mix quinoa with 2 diced apples, 1 cup fresh blueberries, ½ cup chopped walnuts and 1 cup plain non-fat yogurt.

Chicken Quesadillas – heat a medium whole wheat tortilla in a pan, top with cooked shredded chicken, chopped bell pepper (red, green or yellow), shredded low-fat cheese, fresh spinach leaves and a small amount of guacamole; fold over and heat until tortilla is lightly browned then flip and brown the other side.

Simple Salmon – you don't need to do much to salmon to enhance its flavor, keep it simple by seasoning it with salt and pepper then cook it in a small amount of olive oil in a hot pan and squeeze some lime juice over it while cooking.

Tomatoes and Olive Oil – heat some sliced tomatoes in a small amount of olive oil with some basil; serve with a thin slice of mozzarella on top.

Sesame Kale – heat four cloves of minced garlic, one tbsp. minced ginger and 1 tsp. sesame oil in a pan; add 2 tbsp. water and 1 bunch of kale (stemmed and chopped). Cover and cook about 3 minutes; drain then top with 1 tsp. soy sauce and 1 tbsp. sesame seeds.

Swiss chard – sauté chard with a little olive oil and garlic for a simple side dish.

Baked Sweet Potato Fries – cut 2 sweet potatoes into slices, toss with olive oil and paprika; spread on baking sheet and bake for about 15 minutes at 350 degrees then turn and bake for another 10 minutes until lightly crisp.

Power Snack – mix 1 cup chopped walnuts with ½ cup blueberries (fresh or dried) and ¼ cup chunks of dark chocolate.

Yogurt Treat – slice a banana into yogurt and sprinkle with cinnamon.

Tomato Avocado Crisps – using crispbread crackers (like Wasa) top with a mixture of mashed avocado and sun-dried tomatoes; season with salt, pepper and seasonings of choice. Great as a snack or appetizer.

Egg Salad Crisps – similar to above but topping the crispbread with a mixture of chopped hard-boiled eggs, olive oil mayonnaise, Dijon mustard with sea salt and pepper.

Chickpea & Tomato Toss – combine chopped tomato with chickpeas, chopped green onion with a little red wine vinegar and olive oil. Season with garlic powder, salt and pepper.

Simple Snack – mix some cherries or raspberries with nuts like cashews or pistachios.

Banana S'more – top a whole grain graham cracker with some mashed banana and a square of dark chocolate then microwave for 10 seconds until chocolate is slightly melted.

Chapter 6: Starting the Day

After going several hours without food or water while sleeping, your body needs fuel in the morning. Drink water as soon as wake up, before you brush your teeth to rehydrate. Then within an hour or so after waking up refuel your body. Start with a breakfast high in protein and fiber to keep you full and give you the energy needed.

Here are some quick and easy breakfasts for the workdays or when time is limited:

> One hard-boiled egg with a slice of wheat toast and/or with apple slices (or some other type of fruit like berries or melon).

> Oatmeal (sprinkle some cinnamon on top) and some fruit. Or some instant steel cut oats with nuts and raisins or berries.

> Cereal (whole grain/whole wheat); add some blueberries and almonds, sprinkle with cinnamon with skim milk or almond milk.

> Microwave Scramble Eggs: in a large mug or bowl lightly sprayed with nonstick spray whisk 2 eggs (or you can use an egg substitute), add a splash of skim milk and microwave for one minute stirring half way (eggs will rise as they cook). For extra flavor add some chopped onion, turkey bacon bits, low fat cheese, spinach, salsa, etc.

Veggie Scrambled Eggs: coat a pan with low fat cooking spray, sauté some chopped vegetables such as peppers, onions, broccoli, tomatoes, and/or spinach; whisk 2 eggs then add to the vegetable mixture and scramble. Options: add some Pico de Gallo or some feta cheese.

Healthy Omelet: sauté onions, tomatoes, spinach or veggies of choice; whisk 1 egg and 2 egg whites then pour over sautéed veggies and let set lifting the sides so the liquid egg can run underneath. Add some feta cheese then fold over and cook both sides over medium-low heat.

Breakfast tacos: scramble 2 egg whites and 1 whole egg with some green onion; in 2 corn tortillas add the scrambled eggs and top with some salsa and avocado.

Whole wheat waffle (or toast) topped with your choice of yogurt and fruit or spread on some almond butter then drizzle with syrup and top with sliced banana.

A protein shake using a protein powder that is low in sugar made with water and ice or skim milk and adding a fruit of your choice or a smoothie made with yogurt, skim milk and a couple fruit selections.

Two low fat cheese sticks with apple slices.

Cottage-Apple Cheese: mix a cup of low fat cottage cheese with ¼ cup applesauce (unsweetened) with ¼ cup raisins and top with a sprinkle of cinnamon.

Morning or anytime fruit smoothie – in a blender add some frozen mango and frozen strawberries; then add half orange juice and half cranberry juice (preferably low sugar varieties for both juices) so that the liquids are the same level as the fruit. Then add 4-5 ice cubes and blend.

A half cup of low-sugar yogurt (or Greek yogurt) with some granola and topped with fruit such as peach slices then sprinkle with cinnamon.

Whole wheat English muffin topped with peanut or almond butter with slices of banana or berries.

*Watch your portions and read labels; the amount of calories on the above depends on how much you use.

Typically I will have the same thing for breakfast Monday through Friday (something simple) such as a hard-boiled egg and slice of toast; then cook something on Saturday and Sunday. Then the next week I choose something different such as a bowl of organic whole wheat cereal with nuts and fruit and have that Monday through Friday. By having the same thing during the week when time is usually limited I never skip breakfast and feel full until lunch, plus have energy while keeping my calories in the morning in check.

And I love cinnamon, I sprinkle it on my buttered toast, on my toast or waffle with almond butter, on my oatmeal, on my cereal, on my fruit...you get the point, adding cinnamon gives it a "sweet" flavor but much better for you than sugar.

For the weekends or when you have more time to cook, on the following pages are some delicious recipes under 300 calories per serving:

Open-Faced Egg, Bacon and Cheese Sandwich

2 servings

2 slices whole wheat or whole grain bread
1 tsp olive oil
2 eggs
2 wedges of light Swiss cheese (such as Laughing Cow)
2 tbsp turkey bacon bits

Toast the bread in toaster; meanwhile, heat olive oil in a pan over medium heat. Fry the eggs in the oil breaking the yolk and season with a dash of salt and pepper.

On the toast spread each with a wedge of the cheese, sprinkle the turkey bacon bits over the cheese then top each with the cooked egg while it's hot.

Other options are to add some spinach leaves over the bacon bits then top with the hot egg; the heat from the egg will soften the spinach leaves. And you could sprinkle a small amount of shredded cheese on top and heat under a broiler for just a couple of minutes to allow cheese to melt.

If you are sprinkle cheese on top then you may want to switch out the wedge of soft cheese with spreading some light mayo with some mustard on the toast (some Dijon mustard will add a little spice).

Breakfast Burrito

2 servings

2 egg whites
1 whole egg
¼ cup shredded light Mexican cheese
¼ cup canned beans – rinsed (such as black or pinto beans)
2 whole wheat tortillas
2 tbsp salsa

Lightly coat pan/skillet with non-stick spray; in a bowl whisk egg whites with a dash of salt and pepper then scramble in the pan.

Divide the scrambled egg whites on the tortillas then top with cheese and beans; fold the bottom on the tortilla then roll to create a burrito. Heat in the microwave about 30 seconds until beans are hot and cheese is melted.

Top each burrito with salsa and a tsp. of light sour cream if desired.

Easy Garden Quiche

4 servings

1 cup chopped fresh broccoli
½ cup chopped onions
½ cup chopped green peppers
1 cup shredded non-fat (or low-fat) cheddar cheese
1 ½ cup skim milk
¾ cup Bisquick
1 tsp salt
¼ tsp pepper
¾ cup egg substitute

Preheat oven to 400 degrees

Lightly spray pie plate with cooking spray. Heat 1 cup water with salt to boiling; add broccoli, cook until tender then drain thoroughly.

Mix broccoli, onion, green pepper and cheese then put in pie plate.

Beat remaining ingredients until smooth for about 15 seconds in blender and pour into pie plate.

Bake until golden brown 35 to 40 minutes. Let stand 5 minutes before cutting.

Vegetable Omelet

2 servings

½ cup sliced mushrooms
½ cup summer squash sliced thin
½ cup zucchini sliced thin
¼ cup chopped red bell pepper
1 tbsp olive oil
4 eggs
¼ tsp garlic powder
½ tsp dried basil leaves
2 tsp grated Parmesan cheese
¼ cup water

Combine vegetables with oil and sauté in a pan over medium heat about 3-4 minutes until vegetables are tender but still crisp then remove from heat.

Whisk together the eggs, garlic, basil, cheese and water then pour half the mixture into a pan lightly coated with butter; cook lifting the edges and tilting the pan to cook the eggs until it is set and no liquid egg is there.

Add half of the vegetable mixture and fold over the omelet continuing to cook on low for another minute on each side.

Repeat above with remaining mixtures to make second omelet.

Scrambled Eggs with Salmon, Asparagus and Goat Cheese

4 servings

1 tbsp butter
6 asparagus stalks, bottoms removed and chopped into pieces
6 whole eggs
2 egg whites
2 tbsp skim milk
4 oz smoked salmon, chopped
¼ cup goat cheese, crumbled

In a large skillet heat butter on medium until it melts then add asparagus and sauté until tender yet crisp; season with a dash of salt and pepper.

Whisk together the eggs and milk adding a dash of salt and pepper then pour into the pan with asparagus.

Reduce to low heat and cook stirring constantly until the eggs begin to set; stir in the goat cheese.

Remove from heat then add the salmon; let sit for a minute then serve.

Mini Frittatas

8 Servings

Cooking Spray
½ cup chopped onion
2/3 cup chopped ham or salmon
1/3 cup (about 1 ½ ounces) shredded reduced-fat cheddar cheese
2 tbsp chopped fresh chives
1/8 tsp dried thyme
1/8 tsp black pepper
4 large egg whites
1 large egg

Preheat oven to 350 degrees

Heat a large nonstick skillet coated with cooking spray over medium-high heat. Add onion; sauté 2 minutes or until crisp-tender. Add ham (or salmon); sauté 3 minutes.

Remove from heat; cool 5 minutes.

Combine remaining ingredients in a large bowl; stir with a whisk. Add ham mixture, stirring with a whisk. Spoon mixture into 24 miniature muffin cups coated with cooking spray.

Bake at 350 degrees for 20 minutes or until set.

Ham, Egg and Cheese Bread Cups

6 Servings

6 slices of whole wheat bread
¼ cup sliced green onions
1 ½ cups Egg Beaters
¼ cup minced fully cooked lean ham
¼ tsp kosher salt
1/8 tsp ground black pepper
¼ cup shredded low-fat sharp cheddar cheese

Preheat oven to 350 degrees

Spray six 6-ounce custard cups or large muffin cups; trim crusts from bread and spray both sides of each slice then place into cups.

Bake 11 to 13 minutes or until lightly browned and toasted.

Spray medium nonstick skillet and place over medium heat; add green onion and cook for about 1 minute. Pour in Egg Beaters then sprinkle ham, salt and pepper evenly over egg.

Cook without stirring until edges and bottom begin to set.

Place equal amounts of egg mixture in bread cups; sprinkle evenly with cheese. Let stand about 2 minutes or until cheese softens.

Green Chili Breakfast Casserole

4 Servings

1 can chopped green chilies
1 ½ cup shredded low-fat cheddar cheese
1 lb turkey or low-fat sausage cooked and crumbled
2 cup egg substitute
1 cup skim milk

Line bottom of square baking dish with green chilies, half of cheese, then another layer of chilies, then sausage and top with cheese.

Refrigerate overnight.

Beat egg substitute and milk then pour over casserole and bake at 400 degrees for 30 minutes.

Egg, Cheese and Sausage Casserole

12 Servings (prep the night before)

12 ounces turkey sausage (or meatless sausage)
2 cups of 1% low-fat milk
2 cups egg substitute
1 tsp dry mustard
¾ tsp salt
½ tsp ground black pepper
¼ tsp ground red pepper
3 large eggs
16 slices of wheat bread
1 cup finely shredded reduced-fat extra-sharp cheddar cheese
¼ tsp paprika

Coat large nonstick skillet with light cooking spray, heat over medium-high heat. Brown sausage in pan, stirring and breaking into crumbles, about 5 minutes. Remove from heat and let cool.

Combine milk with egg substitute, dry mustard, black and red pepper, and eggs in a large bowl then whisk. Trim crusts from bread and cut into 1 inch cubes. Add bread cubes, sausage and cheddar cheese to milk mixture and stir.

Pour into a 13x9 inch baking dish or 3 quart casserole dish coated with cooking spray; spread evenly then cover and refrigerate 8 hours or overnight. When ready to cook, preheat oven to 350 degrees.

Remove casserole from refrigerator, let stand 30 minutes before cooking. Sprinkle paprika over the casserole then bake at 350 for 45 minutes or until set and lightly browned.

Let stand 10 minutes before serving.

Sweet Potato Breakfast Casserole

8 Servings

1 carton (16 oz) egg substitute
½ cup fat free milk
¼ cup light maple syrup
½ tsp salt
Pinch of ground black pepper
3 cups frozen sweet potato cubes
3 turkey sausage patties chopped (or meatless sausage)
1 cup low fat cottage cheese
½ cup shredded reduced-fat cheddar cheese

Preheat oven to 350 degrees; coat a 13x9 inch baking dish with cooking spray.

In a large bowl combine egg substitute, milk, syrup, salt and pepper; then add sweet potatoes, sausage, cottage cheese and a ¼ cup of the shredded cheese, stir.

Pour mixture into baking dish and bake 35 minutes or until set; sprinkle with remaining shredded cheese (1/4 cup) and bake for 5 more minutes or until cheese melts.

Banana Raspberry Pancakes with a Walnut Honey syrup

4 servings

Pancakes
1 and 1/3 cup pancake mix
¼ tsp ground cinnamon
1 cup low fat buttermilk
¼ cup water
1 egg
1 tbsp canola oil
1 tsp vanilla extract
1 large banana, halved lengthwise and cut into thin slices
½ cup fresh raspberries

Walnut Honey syrup
½ cup chopped walnuts
1/3 cup honey
1 tbsp water

In a large bowl combine pancake mix and cinnamon.

In a separate bowl combine buttermilk, water, egg, oil and vanilla extract. Add this mixture to the pancake mix and whisk until smooth; then fold in the banana and set aside.

Prepare the walnut honey syrup by combining the walnuts, honey and water in a bowl, stir.

Coat a large skillet with cooking spray and heat over medium heat; spoon in pancake batter and cook about 2 minutes each side until lightly browned.

Serve with syrup and top with fresh raspberries.

Smoothies

Smoothies are quick and easy to prepare so they make a great breakfast but depending on the smoothie they are great for lunch or as a snack. When adding the ingredients keep an eye on the amount of sugar especially if using yogurt or juices. Here are some favorite smoothie recipes:

Blueberry Smoothie

SERVINGS: 1

1 cup skim milk or unsweetened almond milk
1 cup frozen unsweetened blueberries (or swap out with frozen peaches for a Peach smoothie)
1 tbsp cold-pressed organic flaxseed oil

COMBINE milk and blueberries in blender, and blend for 1 minute. Transfer to glass, and stir in flaxseed oil.

Peanut Butter and Banana Smoothie

SERVINGS: 1

½ cup fat-free milk or plain unsweetened almond milk
½ cup fat-free plain yogurt
2 tbsp creamy natural unsalted peanut butter
¼ very ripe banana
1 tbsp honey
4 ice cubes

COMBINE ingredients in a blender. Process until smooth. Pour into a tall glass and serve.

Chocolate Raspberry Smoothie

SERVINGS: 1

½ cup skim or soy milk
6 oz (80-calorie) vanilla yogurt
¼ cup chocolate chips
1 cup fresh raspberries
Handful of ice OR 1 cup frozen raspberries

COMBINE ingredients in a blender. Blend for 1 minute, transfer to a glass, and eat with a spoon.

Lemon-Orange Citrus Smoothie

SERVINGS: 1

1 cup skim or soy milk
6 oz low calorie lemon yogurt
1 med orange peeled, cleaned, and sliced into sections
Handful of ice
1 tbsp flaxseed oil

COMBINE milk, yogurt, orange, and ice in a blender. Blend for 1 minute, transfer to a glass, and stir in flaxseed oil.

Orange Creamsicle Smoothie

SERVINGS: 1

1 navel orange, peeled
¼ cup fat-free half-and-half or fat-free yogurt

2 tbsp frozen orange juice concentrate

¼ tsp vanilla extract

4 ice cubes

COMBINE the orange, half-and-half or yogurt, orange juice concentrate, vanilla, and ice cubes. Process until smooth.

Apple Smoothie

SERVINGS: 1

½ cup skim or soy milk

6 oz low calorie vanilla yogurt

1 tsp apple pie spice

1 med apple peeled and chopped

2 tbsp cashew butter

Handful of ice

COMBINE ingredients in a blender. Blend for 1 minute, transfer to a glass, and eat with a spoon.

Berry Happy Smoothie

SERVINGS: 2

1 cup frozen unsweetened raspberries

¾ cup chilled unsweetened almond milk

¼ cup frozen pitted unsweetened cherries or raspberries

1½ tbsp honey

2 tsp finely grated fresh ginger

1 tsp ground flaxseed

2 tsp fresh lemon juice

COMBINE all ingredients in blender, adding lemon juice to taste. Puree until smooth. Pour into 2 chilled glasses.

Fruity Banana Smoothie

SERVINGS: 1

1 cup plain nonfat yogurt
1 banana
½ cup orange juice
6 frozen strawberries

COMBINE the yogurt, banana, juice, and strawberries for 20 seconds. Scrape down the sides and blend for an additional 15 seconds.

Peachy Green Smoothie

1 cup spinach leaves (or chopped kale)
1 cup frozen peach slices, slightly thawed
½ cup sliced banana
½ cup light vanilla soymilk
One 5.3-oz container (about ½ cup) fat-free vanilla Greek yogurt
½ cup crushed ice *or* 3 - 4 ice cubes

COMBINE all ingredients in a blender. Blend at high speed until smooth. Enjoy!

Super Skinny Smoothie

3 ounces vanilla Greek yogurt
1 tbsp almond butter
½ cup frozen blueberries
½ cup frozen pineapple
1 cup kale
¾ cup water

COMBINE all ingredients in a blender and process until smooth. Drink up!

Tropical Kale Smoothie

½ cup coconut milk
2 cups chopped kale or spinach (remove stems)
1 ½ cups chopped pineapple
1 ripe banana, chopped

COMBINE the coconut milk, ½ cup water, kale, pineapple and banana in blender; process until smooth, about a minute. Add more water if needed to reach desired consistency.

Chapter 7: Lunches and Dinners

Like breakfast, if you work a Monday through Friday full-time job I find it helpful to have the same thing for lunch each week so I'm not trying to figure out each day what to have (and possibly make bad choices). A typical lunch is a Veggie Sandwich (see below) and some fresh fruit or a large salad. Usually lunch is my main meal and dinner is smaller, lighter meal.

Here are some quick and easy items you can put together quickly and easily for lunches or dinner:

Veggie sandwich – two slices of bread such as an organic, whole wheat bread lightly toasted; spread on a little light mayo and some mustard (or Dijon mustard) and top with slices of cucumber, sliced avocado, tomato and some red leaf lettuce (change up the veggies to suit your taste).

Tuna salad sandwich – Mix tuna with tsp. Dijon mustard, tbsp. plain nonfat yogurt or low-fat mayonnaise, small amount of garlic salt, some chopped green onion and a dash of dill and/or chives.

Turkey sandwich – on whole wheat with romaine lettuce, low fat mayo and mustard.

Chicken salad sandwich – mix cubes of chicken breast (can use can of chunk white chicken) with 3 tbsp. reduced-fat mayo, 2 tbsp. reduced-fat sour cream, 1 and ½ tbsp. chopped tarragon, 2 tbsp. chopped almonds, 1 stalk of celery chopped.

Chicken breast sandwich – serve chicken breast on whole wheat with reduced-fat or light mayo, Dijon mustard, romaine lettuce, tomato slice (option: add some sliced avocado and/or pickles).

Curry Chicken Salad Lettuce Cups – mix together chunks of chicken (either chopped cooked chicken breasts or use a can of chicken chunks), chopped celery, chopped red pepper, and chopped tomato with some light mayo, mustard and curry powder. Serve in lettuce cups (leaves).

Spinach wrap – take a large tortilla (whole wheat) and sprinkle some shredded lite cheese such as Mexican flavor or any type of cheese on top of the tortilla; heat under the broiler until cheese melts (just a few minutes) then top with fresh spinach and sprinkle in some bacon bits. Drizzle some red wine vinegar over it then roll into a wrap. You will be surprised at how good this is! And kids love it!

Sides with your sandwich: side salad, carrot sticks or celery with low fat dip, fruit salad or fruit chunks, apple slices, low fat yogurt.

Roast Beef Roll-Up – on a whole wheat tortilla spread 2 tbsp. of light cream cheese or 1 wedge of light Swiss cheese; then top with thinly sliced roast beef, 2 tbsp. of deli mustard and lettuce then roll up.

Lunch salad with mixed leafy greens, a variety of veggies, topped with turkey and chopped egg whites, then dress with a mixture of flaxseed oil and balsamic vinegar. Also by adding your favorite herbs such as cilantro, rosemary, mint or basil it will add spice to your salad so you can get by with less dressing.

Garbanzo Salad – combine a bag of broccoli slaw with a can of garbanzo beans, drained and rinsed; add 1/3 cup of Italian dressing and stir to coat. Add some turkey pepperoni and feta cheese.

Quinoa with veggies – cook quinoa for either 2, 4 or 6 servings if you want to make extra since it keeps well and you can use it over 2 or 3 days; sauté some chopped asparagus with garlic in some light olive oil then combine with the quinoa; then add some crumbled feta cheese. You could add other veggies such as tomatoes, onions, spinach or broccoli instead of asparagus, etc.

Soup and salad – choose an organic soup that is low in fat and sodium and serve with a side salad.

Spinach Salad – ¼ cup pecans, 1 chopped pear and 2 cups baby spinach with ¼ cup feta cheese and 1 tbsp. light raspberry vinaigrette.

Spring Salad – ¼ cup walnuts, 1 chopped apple, and 2 cups spring mix salad with 1 tbsp. sesame seeds topped with 1 tsp. olive oil and 1 tsp. balsamic vinegar.

Arugula Chicken Salad – add to baby arugula some grated parmesan cheese, diced chicken breast, virgin olive oil and fresh lemon juice then toss.

Tortilla Soup – in chicken broth add some sliced or diced chicken breast, chopped white onion, diced tomatoes and avocado; top with a few pieces of tortilla chips. Make a large amount ahead by leaving out the avocado and tortilla chips then add those when you serve.

Mini Personal Pizzas – Top four mini whole wheat pita with a tablespoon of marinara sauce on each (all natural preferred), then top with shredded part-skim mozzarella, chopped fresh tomatoes, and chopped fresh basil. Cook under the broiler until cheese melts. Serves 2 for lunch or prepare several to serve as appetizers. For a variation of flavor top with cheese, tomatoes and crumbled turkey bacon.

Mexican Rice Casserole – in a microwave safe casserole dish cook brown rice according to instructions on the box and for the amount of servings you choose; heat up a can of black beans (optional: add taco seasoning to beans), drain then add the beans to the cooked brown rice (season rice to taste with salt and pepper or other seasoning of choice). Add some salsa or Pico de Gallo and a small amount of shredded reduced-fat Mexican cheese and mix together. Serve with a small amount of guacamole and low-fat sour cream if desired.

Quick Quesadilla – spread a wedge of Laughing Cow cheese wedge over a whole-wheat tortilla then heat in a large pan over medium heat; sprinkle on the tortilla ¼ cup diced cooked chicken, 1 tbsp. chopped fresh cilantro and a tbsp. of salsa. After a minute or two when flip the tortilla over in half and cook for about a minute then flip over and cook for another minute.

Twice-baked Mexican Potato – puncture potato with fork and cook in microwave (usually 6-8 minutes but microwaves vary); once the potato cools, scoop out the inside and put in a small bowl. Combine with salsa then add back into the shell; sprinkle low-fat shredded Mexican cheese over the top and bake for about 10 minutes at 375 degrees until hot and cheese is melted. Serve with scallions and low-fat sour cream if desired.

Pasta with Broccoli, Beans and Feta – toss together 1 cup whole wheat penne pasta (cooked), 1 ounce feta cheese, ½ cup cannellini beans, and one cup chopped broccoli and 2 tsp. olive oil.

Simple Chicken Pasta – mix 2 cups cooked whole wheat rotini, 1/3 cup sundried tomatoes or fresh diced tomatoes, ½ cup chicken broth, minced garlic, 1 tbsp. olive oil and a cup of cooked chicken breast.

Simple Cheesy Pasta – mix cooked whole wheat penne (or pasta of choice), drained and still hot, with some light butter and crumbled goat cheese. The cheese will melt as stirred, season with sea salt and pepper.

Veggie Pasta – in a pan heat a tbsp. of olive oil with some garlic and basil, then using a bag of broccoli slaw add some to the pan and sauté for a few minutes; then stir in some marinara sauce until heated through and top with Mediterranean style crumbled-feta cheese or some shredded mozzarella. You can also add this to some real pasta for a heartier meal but limiting the amount of pasta needed.

In a pinch for something quick and easy for lunch, have some instant oatmeal with fruit and nuts; or a peanut butter sandwich on whole wheat with an apple.

Plan your meals using smart food choices; here are some of the best choices to make when choosing ingredients:

Proteins:

- Beans such as black, garbanzo, kidney or lentils
- Low-fat or fat-free cheese
- Skinless chicken or turkey breast
- Eggs
- Tofu
- Beans
- Fish such as salmon, sole, flounder
- Shellfish such as shrimp, lobster, crab

Vegetables:

- Steamed fresh vegetables such as broccoli, cauliflower, asparagus, zucchini, squash, sugarsnap peas, artichoke, Brussels sprouts
- Raw fresh vegetables such as broccoli, cauliflower, cucumber, celery, radishes, zucchini, peppers

- Dark leafy salad greens such as spinach, arugula, spring mix

Starches/Breads:

- Whole-wheat, rye, multigrain bread
- High fiber, low sugar cereal
- Oatmeal
- Whole-wheat pasta
- Brown rice
- Sweet potato
- Quinoa

Fruits:

- Apple or pears
- Berries such as strawberries, blueberries, raspberries, blackberries
- Grapefruit
- Fresh melon such as cantaloupe or honeydew

Fats:

- Almonds
- Avocado
- Olive oil
- Peanut or almond butter
- Oil and vinegar salad dressing, add lemon, lime or mustard

When you have time to cook, here are some delicious recipes under 500 calories per serving (sides are in the next chapter):

Chicken Stroganoff

4 Servings

4 slices of turkey-bacon
1 pound skinless, boneless chicken breasts, cut into strips
½ tsp salt
¼ tsp paprika
1 container (8 ounce) reduced-fat sour cream
4 cups hot cooked medium egg noodles
1 ½ cups chopped onion
1 ½ cups fat-free, low-sodium chicken broth
½ tsp pepper
2 cloves minced garlic
2 tbsp flour

Cook bacon in a large nonstick skillet over medium heat until crisp; once cooled crumble bacon. Add onion and chicken to bacon drippings in pan, sauté 6 minutes.

Add bacon, broth, salt, pepper, paprika, and garlic then bring to a boil.

Cover, reduce heat and simmer for 10 minutes. In a bowl combine sour cream and flour, stir until smooth.

Add sour cream mixture to pan then bring to a boil. Reduce heat and simmer 2 minutes, stirring constantly. Serve over egg noodles.

Italian Chicken Pasta

4 Servings

6 oz of whole wheat noodle pasta (about ½ a package)
3 cups marinara sauce
2 cups chopped cooked chicken breast
2 cups shredded mozzarella cheese
¼ cup grated parmesan cheese

Heat oven to 375 degrees; cook pasta according to package directions.

Meanwhile, heat marinara sauce and chicken in saucepan until warm.

In a 2 quart casserole dish, spoon sauce mixture over bottom then layer with half the pasta and sprinkle half the mozzarella cheese; follow with another layer of chicken/sauce and repeat with remaining pasta and mozzarella. Top with parmesan cheese.

Bake uncovered for 20 minutes or until hot and bubbly.

Rosemary Chicken Couscous Salad

2 Servings

2 cups chicken broth
1 (10 ounce) box couscous
¾ cup olive oil
¼ cup fresh lemon juice
2 tbsp white balsamic vinegar
¼ cup chopped fresh rosemary leaves
Salt and ground black pepper to taste
2 large cooked skinless, boneless chicken breast halves, cut
into bite-size pieces
1 cup chopped English cucumber
½ cup chopped sun-dried tomatoes
½ cup chopped pitted Kalamata olives
½ cup crumbled feta cheese
¼ cup chopped fresh Italian parsley salt and ground black
pepper to taste

Place chicken stock in a saucepan and bring to a boil over
medium-high heat. Stir in couscous. Remove pan from the
heat; cover, and let stand for 5 minutes. Fluff couscous with
a fork. Cool for 10 minutes.

Meanwhile, make the dressing by combining the olive oil,
lemon juice, and vinegar in the bowl of a blender or food
processor; mix on low until mixture thickens. Stir in
rosemary. Season to taste with salt and pepper.

Combine the chicken, cucumber, sun-dried tomatoes, and
olives in a large bowl. Stir in the couscous, Feta cheese, and
parsley. Season to taste with salt and pepper. Toss the salad
with half the dressing. Taste, and add more dressing as
desired, or, if making the salad in advance, add additional
dressing just before serving.

Quick and Easy Polynesian Chicken

4 Servings

1 tablespoon plus 1 teaspoon olive oil
4 Boneless chicken breasts
1 can crushed pineapple
Small jar of peach or apricot preserves (low sugar)

Heat olive oil in a large nonstick skillet over medium-high heat. Add chicken and sauté about three minutes on each side.

Mix together the can of crushed pineapple (with juice) and preserves then pour over chicken; reduce heat, cover and simmer about 20 minutes.

Serve with brown rice and a vegetable side or salad.

Greek Chicken in a Tomato Sauce

4 Servings

1 tbsp olive oil
2 cups chopped red onion
1 cup chopped yellow bell pepper
4 tbsp lemon juice
1 tsp dried basil
2 cans diced tomatoes in garlic and olive oil
4 Boneless chicken breasts
Crumbled Feta cheese

Heat olive oil in a large nonstick skillet over medium-high heat. Add chicken to pan and sauté about three minutes on each side.

Add onion, peppers, lemon juice, basil and cans of tomatoes to pan; stir well.

Cover, reduce heat, and simmer about 25 minutes until chicken is done.

Serve over angel hair pasta, brown rice or quinoa. Sprinkle feta cheese on top.

Southwest Chicken Cutlets

2 Servings

2 boneless chicken cutlets; pounded to about ½ inch
thickness
2 tbsp of light cream cheese or 2 wedges of Laughing Cow
Light Swiss Cheese
¼ cup salsa
¼ cup green onion, chopped

Preheat oven to 350 degrees.

Season chicken cutlets with a little salt and pepper; spread
on each cutlet the creamy cheese then top evenly with salsa
and the chopped green onion.

Roll each cutlet up, secure with a toothpick and place in a
baking dish which has been sprayed with non-stick spray.

Cover with aluminum foil and bake for 20 minutes.

Remove foil then bake for another 15 minutes until chicken
is cooked through.

Suggested side: Mexican rice or black beans.

Italian Chicken Packets

2 Servings

2 cups chopped broccoli (frozen)
2 boneless skinless chicken breast
½ cup diced tomatoes
¼ cup light Italian dressing

Preheat oven to 450 degrees.

Combine broccoli, tomatoes and Italian dressing in bowl.

For packet lay out 2 large sheets of heavy-duty foil. Place one chicken breast on each piece of foil and spread broccoli mixture equally over each chicken breast then fold over and seal foil leaving some space for steam.

Place packets on baking sheet and bake for 20-25 minutes until chicken is cooked.

Herb-Crusted Pork Tenderloin

4 Servings

1 pound pork tenderloin
2 tsp olive oil
1 tsp sage
1 tsp thyme
½ tsp minced garlic
¼ tsp ground black pepper
Salt and pepper

Preheat oven to 375 degrees.

Cover a baking sheet and with aluminum foil and place pork on the pan. Drizzle oil over pork and sprinkle with sage, thyme, garlic, pepper and salt to taste. Rub to coat evenly.

Place in oven and roast until the meat reaches 155 degrees and the juices run clear, about 30-35 minutes.

Let stand 10 minutes before slicing.

Serve with sautéed new potatoes and a steamed vegetable.

Spicy Pork Cutlets

2 Servings

One 8oz pork tenderloin, cut into 4 rounds
½ tsp chili powder
2 tsp olive oil
¼ cup baby carrots, sliced or julienned
½ tsp minced garlic

With a scaloppini pounder or rolling pin covered in plastic, pound pork to flatten to about ½ inch thickness.

Season both sides with chili powder and salt to taste.

Heat oil in skillet on high for about 1 minute; add pork and cook until browned, about 1 minute each side. Add carrots and garlic then reduce heat to medium.

Cover and cook, stirring occasionally, until pork is no longer pink and juices run clear, about 5 minutes.

Serve with cauliflower mash.

Turkey Meatloaf

6-8 Servings

1 tbsp olive oil
2 stalks celery, finely chopped
1 small onion, finely chopped
1 clove garlic, minced
2 lbs ground turkey
¾ cup whole wheat bread crumbs
1/3 cup skim milk
1 tbsp Worcestershire sauce
2 egg whites
½ cup ketchup (low sugar)
½ tsp salt
¼ tsp pepper
1 tbsp Dijon mustard

Preheat oven to 350 degrees.

In a large skillet add oil, celery and onion and cook over medium heat until softened; add garlic and cook for about one more minute. Transfer to a bowl and let cool.

Once the vegetable mixture is cool add turkey, bread crumbs, milk Worcestershire sauce, egg, ¼ cup ketchup salt and pepper; mix together with hands then shape into a loaf and place in a metal baking pan.

In a separate small bowl mix the remaining ¼ cup of ketchup with Dijon mustard then spread over the loaf.

Bake for 60 minutes then let stand for 10 minutes before serving.

Serve with cauliflower mash.

Honey-Mustard Turkey Tenders

4 Servings

14 oz. turkey breast tenders (boneless, skinless)
2 tsp olive oil
2 tsp Dijon mustard
1 tbsp honey

Preheat oven to 375 degrees.

Cover the top of baking sheet with aluminum foil then place turkey breast tenders on the foil in the center.

In a small bowl, mix the oil, mustard and honey then drizzle over the turkey and rotate to coat evenly. Then fold the foil to create a packet and seal the seams tight but keeping the foil loose around the tenders.

Bake until the turkey reaches 165 degrees and until juices run clear, about 30 minutes.

Carefully unwrap foil and flip the tenders over then allow to sit about another 10 minutes.

Suggested sides: new potatoes or a side salad.

Grilled Lime Tuna Steak

4 Servings

¼ cup olive oil
1 tsp celery salt
1 tsp paprika
1 tsp black pepper
2 tsp cilantro
2 limes
1 pound tuna steaks

Combine all the ingredients except for the tuna in a shallow dish; then coat both sides of the tuna steaks with the mixture and refrigerate for 20 minutes turning occasionally.

Broil or grill the steaks 8-10 minutes per inch of thickness or until the tuna flakes easily with a fork.

Suggested sides: sautéed new potatoes with a vegetable or with brown rice with peas and onions.

.

Halibut with Tomatoes and Capers

4 Servings

1 tablespoon plus 1 teaspoon olive oil
2 cloves garlic, sliced
1 pint grape tomatoes cut in half
½ cup fresh orange juice
½ cup fresh flat-leaf parsley
2 tbsp capers
Salt and pepper
4 – 6 ounce pieces of skinless halibut fillet or some other
firm-fleshed white fish

Heat 1 tablespoon of the oil in a large skillet over medium-high heat; add the garlic and cook, stirring often for about 30 seconds. Add the tomatoes, orange juice, parsley, capers, ½ tsp. salt, and ¼ tsp. pepper, simmer until some of the tomatoes begin to break down (about 4-5 minutes).

Meanwhile, heat the remaining teaspoon of oil in a large nonstick skillet over medium-high heat; season the fish with ¼ tsp. each of salt and pepper.

Cook until opaque throughout, 3 to 5 minutes per side.

Serve with the tomatoes.

Garlic Shrimp with paprika

6 Servings

1 ½ pounds large shrimp (20-25 per pound), peeled and
deveined with tails on
2 tbsp olive oil
1 tbsp smoked paprika
1 tsp garlic powder
1/8 tsp cayenne pepper
¾ tsp salt

Preheat oven to 425 degrees. Spray a baking sheet with
cooking spray.

Rinse shrimp and dry well with paper towel.

In a large bowl, mix together oil, paprika, garlic powder, salt
and cayenne; add the shrimp and toss to coat evenly.

Place the baking sheet in the oven for 4 minutes to preheat
it then place the shrimp on the hot baking sheet and cook
for 6 minutes; then turn and cook for about another 4
minutes until the shrimp is opaque in the center.

Suggested sides: serve with whole wheat pasta and spinach

Healthy Shrimp Scampi

2 Servings

1 tsp olive oil
1 clove garlic, crushed
½ tsp dried basil
½ cup chopped spinach leaves
20-24 large frozen shrimp (peeled and deveined)
Splash of hot sauce
Sesame seeds (optional)

In a large bowl, mix all the ingredients tossing well to coat the shrimp.

Spray a large pan with non-stick spray and add the shrimp mixture; sauté over medium heat until shrimp is opaque.

Sprinkle top with sesame seeds if desired.

Serve with whole wheat pasta or brown rice.

Grilled Salmon with Cucumber Salad

4 Servings

4 salmon filets or salmon steaks
1 tsp olive oil
Salt and pepper
¼ cup nonfat Greek yogurt
1 tbsp white wine vinegar
2 cucumbers, thinly sliced
2 stalks of celery, thinly sliced
¼ cup fresh parsley

In a large bowl, mix together yogurt, vinegar, and about a ¼ teaspoon of salt and pepper; add cucumbers, celery and parsley then toss to mix. Refrigerate while grilling the salmon.

Season salmon with salt and pepper then grill over medium-high heat until opaque, about 5 to 6 minutes per side depending on the thickness.

Serve with cucumber salad.

Roasted Salmon and Potatoes

4 Servings

3 tbsp olive oil
1 pound new potatoes (about 10 small ones), halved
2 scallions, chopped
Salt and pepper
16 oz salmon fillet
1 tbsp red wine vinegar
1 tbsp whole-grain mustard
1 tsp honey
2 tbsp fresh parsley, chopped

Heat oven to 400 degrees; on a baking sheet toss the potatoes, scallions, 1 tablespoon of the olive oil and a ½ teaspoon each of salt and pepper.

Roast in the oven, tossing half way through, until the potatoes begin to soften, about 20 minutes total.

Then push the potatoes around the sides and place the salmon fillet in the center. Season with ¼ teaspoon each of salt and pepper and roast about 12 – 15 minutes until the salmon is opaque and the potatoes are golden brown.

Meanwhile, in a bowl, combine the vinegar, mustard, honey, parsley, the remaining 2 tablespoons of olive oil and ¼ teaspoon each salt and pepper, whisk together. Drizzle the mixture over the salmon and potatoes.

Spicy Barbeque Salmon

1 Serving

2 tbsp BBQ sauce with 45 calories or less per 2-tbsp. serving
1 tsp Sriracha sauce
1 cup broccoli florets
½ cup chopped yellow squash
½ cup chopped zucchini
One 4-oz raw skinless salmon fillet

Directions:
Preheat oven to 375 degrees. Lay a large piece of heavy-duty foil on a baking sheet and spray with nonstick spray.

In a small bowl, mix BBQ sauce with Sriracha sauce until uniform.

Lay veggies on the center of the foil. Top with salmon and drizzle with sauce mixture. Cover with another large piece of foil.

Fold together and seal all four edges of the foil pieces, forming a well-sealed packet. Bake for 20 minutes, or until veggies are tender and fish is cooked through.

Allow packet to cool for a few minutes, and then cut to release steam before opening it entirely. (Careful -- steam will be hot.)

Grilled Salmon with Pineapple Salsa

4 Servings

Salsa:
2 cups diced pineapple
¼ cup diced red onion
1 diced red bell pepper
¼ cup fresh minced cilantro
2 limes

Prepare salsa at least 4-5 hours in advance; combine all ingredients in small bowl then refrigerate.

4 salmon filets
2 teaspoon olive oil
Dash of salt and pepper

Brush olive oil on salmon then season with salt and pepper; place salmon skin side up on grill and cook for about 5 minutes then turn and grill for about another 5 minutes until opaque.

Top with salsa.

Skillet Tilapia with Black Beans & Kale

2 Servings

2 tbsp chopped red onion
1 tbsp olive oil
1 tsp crushed fennel seeds
1 cup chopped kale leaves
½ cup rinsed and drained canned black beans
2 tilapia fillets
   Paprika for garnish
2 lemon wedges

In a skillet, combine onion, oil, fennel and salt to taste. Cook over medium heat, stirring occasionally until softened, about 5 minutes.

Then add kale and stir to coat with seasonings; cook until kale starts to wilt, about 2 minutes. Stir in beans; set tilapia on mixture and dust lightly with paprika.

Cover and cook until tilapia is cooked through, about 10 minutes.

Serve with lemon wedges.

Crumb Topped Tilapia

4 Servings

4 tbsp bread crumbs
1 tsp oregano
½ tsp minced garlic
2 tbsp olive oil
4 tilapia fillets
4 lemon wedges for garnish

Preheat oven to 375 degrees.

Combine bread crumbs, oregano, garlic and a pinch of salt in a bowl. On the tilapia fillets drizzle half of the olive oil (or 1 tbsp.); then rub the bread crumb mixture around each filet to coat. Drizzle the remaining oil over the coated fillets.

Bake tilapia about 10 minutes until cooked through.

Serve with lemon wedges.

Butternut Squash Mac-n-Cheese

6 Servings

2 ½ pounds butternut squash, peeled, halved, and seeded,
then quartered and sliced into triangles
6 garlic cloves
1 thyme sprig
2 cups unsweetened almond milk
2 cups chicken stock, or vegetable stock
1 pound small elbow macaroni or mini shells
2 tbsp grated Gruyere

Herbed breadcrumb topping:
¾ cup panko breadcrumbs
1 tbsp finely chopped flat-leaf parsley
2 garlic cloves, minced
¼ tsp sea salt

Preheat the oven to 375°F.
In a large saucepan, add the squash, garlic cloves, thyme
sprig, unsweetened almond milk, and stock. Cook until the
squash is fork-tender. Remove the sprig of thyme.
Place the squash mixture in a food processor or blender and
puree until velvety smooth.
Cook macaroni in salted water until it is al dente. Drain and
rinse with cool water. Spread out the macaroni in a lightly
greased 13-inch x 9-inch pan. Pour the squash puree over
the noodles.
To make the breadcrumbs and bake
Combine all the ingredients for the herbed breadcrumb
topping. Cover the mac 'n' cheese with foil and bake
approximately 45 minutes. Remove from the oven and
evenly spread the breadcrumb topping and Gruyere over
the top. Transfer to the broiler and broil for 5 to 10 minutes,
or until the cheese is brown and bubbly.

Slow Cooker Organic Bean Stew

4 – 6 Servings

1 carton organic vegetable broth
1 can organic black beans
1 can organic garbanzo beans
1 can organic kidney beans
2 cans organic tomato sauce
1 head of cabbage (chopped)
8 medium carrots (chopped)
2 tsp organic Adobo seasoning
½ tsp organic garlic powder
½ tsp sea salt

Add broth, black beans, garbanzo beans, kidney beans and tomato sauce to slow cooker. Then add Adobo seasoning, garlic powder and sea salt.

Finally, add vegetables; stir mixture to combine.

Cook on high for 4-5 hours

Vegan Avocado Pasta

3 Servings

9 oz (255 g) uncooked pasta (use gluten-free, if desired)
1 to 2 cloves garlic, to taste
¼ cup (60 mL) fresh basil leaves, plus more for serving
4 to 6 tsp (20 to 30 mL) fresh lemon juice, to taste
1 tbsp (15 mL) extra-virgin olive oil
1 ripe medium avocado, pitted
¼ to ½ tsp (1 to 2 mL) fine-grain sea salt
Freshly ground black pepper
Lemon zest, for serving

Bring a large pot of salted water to a boil. Cook pasta according to the instructions on the package.

Make the sauce while pasta cooks: In a food processor, combine garlic and basil and pulse to mince. Add lemon juice, oil, avocado flesh, and 1 tbsp. (15 mL) water, and process until smooth, stopping to scrape down the bowl as needed. If sauce is too thick, add another 1 tbsp. (15 mL) water. Season with salt and pepper to taste.

Drain pasta and place it back in the pot. Add the avocado sauce and stir until combined. You can gently rewarm the pasta if it has cooled slightly, or simply serve at room temperature.
Top with lemon zest, pepper, and fresh basil leaves, if desired.

Black Bean Cakes

4 Servings

1 cup canned black beans, rinsed and drained
¼ cup cooked herb rice pilaf (cold)
¼ cup bread crumbs
2 tbsp finely chopped broccoli florets (cooked)
1 egg white
½ tsp minced garlic
¼ tsp paprika
4 tsp crumbled feta cheese

Combine all ingredients except for the feta cheese in a food processor; pulse until mixture is coarsely ground and sticky. Divide the mixture into four patties.

Preheat skillet over medium heat about one minute; coat with non-stick cooking spray.

Cook patties for two minutes on each side until browned.

Sprinkle feta over the top of each cake then cover skillet for about a minute while the cheese melts.

Suggested sides: new potatoes or a side salad.

SALADS

Black Bean Salad

4 Servings

¼ cup tomato vinaigrette
1 can black beans, drained
1 tsp ground cumin
2 cups corn, preferably fresh kernels (if using frozen be sure to thaw and dry)
2 oz smoked mozzarella, diced
1 pint cherry tomatoes, quartered
¾ cup chopped avocado
½ cup red onion (finely chopped)
¼ cup fresh cilantro, chopped

Combine vinaigrette, beans, cumin, with a dash of salt and pepper and set aside.

Heat a large skillet over medium-high heat; add corn and sauté stirring occasionally until lightly browned (about 3-4 minutes).

Let the corn cool then add to the bean mixture along with the rest of the ingredients and mix together.

Chill for about 30 minutes then serve.

Green Salad with Turkey

4 Servings

2 tbsp balsamic vinegar
1 tsp Dijon mustard
3 tbsp olive oil
8 cups field greens or spring mix
12 oz of cubed roasted turkey
1 ½ cup yellow bell pepper, julienned
1 cup dried cranberries
½ cup thinly sliced red onion

Combine vinegar and mustard in a small bowl then whisk in olive oil with salt and pepper, set aside.

In a large bowl combine greens, turkey, bell pepper, cranberries and onion, toss together.

When ready to serve, toss vinaigrette with salad mixture.

Apple Walnut Salad

4 Servings

4 cups spring mix greens
4 apples, cored and chopped
1 cup chopped walnuts
½ cup gorgonzola cheese
¼ cup champagne vinaigrette or blush wine vinaigrette

In a large bowl combine the spring mix, apples and walnuts then toss with dressing.

Sprinkle gorgonzola cheese evenly on top.

Serve as a main dish or with grilled chicken.

Avocado Citrus Salad

6 Servings

8 cups mixed salad greens
2 oranges, separated into segments and chopped
1 firm avocado, chopped
1 tbsp chopped walnuts

Place greens in large bowl and add oranges, walnuts and avocado.

For dressing mix together:

2 tbsp. lime juice
2 tbsp. olive oil
1 tbsp. finely chopped cilantro
¼ tsp. salt
1/8 tsp. ground black or red pepper

Strawberry Peach Chicken Salad

4 Servings

6 cups spring or mixed salad greens
1 lb cooked boneless, skinless chicken breast cut into strips
1 cup sliced strawberries
1 peach, peeled and sliced
2 green onions, chopped

Dressing:
1 cup fat-free strawberry yogurt
1 cup sliced strawberries
2 tbsp red wine vinegar

Mix greens, strawberries, peach and green onions; top with chicken breast.

For dressing place ingredients in a blender or food processor and blend for about 20 seconds or until smooth.

Top salad with the dressing.

Garbanzo Bean Salad

2 Servings

1 can (6 oz) garbanzo beans, drained
1 oz shredded Swiss cheese (or other cheese of choice)
1 diced tomato
¼ cup sliced green onion
1 tbsp parsley
1 tbsp olive oil and 1 tbsp. lemon juice
½ clove garlic, minced
¼ tsp each of salt and pepper
4-6 romaine hearts (inner leaves of romaine lettuce)
1 hard-boiled egg, cut into quarters

In a bowl combine garbanzo beans, shredded cheese, tomato, onions, and parsley.

In a separate bowl combine oil, lemon juice, garlic, salt and pepper; mix then pour over bean mixture and toss together.

Serve over romaine lettuce and top with egg.

Shrimp and Cabbage Salad

4 Servings

1 head of cabbage shredded (or bag of pre-shredded cabbage)
¾ pound of cooked medium shrimp (shelled, deveined and no-tail)
½ cup diced onion
½ cup chopped green bell pepper
3 tbsp low-fat sour cream
2 tbsp chili sauce
1 ½ tbsp low-fat mayonnaise
1 tbsp horseradish sauce
1 tsp sugar
Dash of pepper

Combine in a large bowl the cabbage, shrimp, onion and bell pepper and let chill in refrigerator.

Then combine the remaining ingredients in another bowl for the dressing and chill for about 30 minutes.

To serve pour the dressing over the cabbage/shrimp salad and toss; serve with a lemon wedge as garnish.

Veggie Tuna Salad

4 Servings

One 12-oz can or pouch albacore tuna packed in water, drained and flaked
1 cup finely chopped red and yellow bell peppers
½ cup finely chopped carrots
½ cup finely chopped celery
2/3 cup fat-free mayonnaise
1 tbsp plus 1 tsp. honey mustard
2 tsp sweet relish
1/8 tsp salt, or more to taste
1/8 tsp black pepper, or more to taste

Combine in a large bowl the tuna with the other ingredients and mix well; change it up by swapping the honey mustard for a spicy mustard or other flavored mustards.

Serve on top a spring mix or arugula salad with some balsamic vinegar and/or lemon wedges.

Chapter 8: Snacks, Apps and Sides

Here are some quick and easy suggestions for snacks and some can be used as a side:

A cup of nonfat plain Greek yogurt; add a teaspoon of almond butter and add honey to taste (not too much though) then stir; it's a delicious creamy snack or add some banana or fruit for a dessert.

Apple slices with almond butter (add celery for variation) or apple slices with Laughing Cow Light Swiss cream cheese (optional: add some whole wheat crackers).

Make yourself a plate with grapes, some low fat cheese slices and a few whole wheat crackers.

Cucumber slices and/or carrot sticks with: hummus, light cream cheese or plain (maybe with a little salt and pepper on the cucumber slices).

Fruit such as grapes, strawberries, blueberries, watermelon, pears, and grapefruit...all make great snacks.

A mini-bag of popcorn lightly with a light spritz of butter.

Handful of almonds or pistachios.

12 raw cashews and 8 medium strawberries.

20 raw almonds with ½ cup unsweetened applesauce.

½ cup Greek yogurt with 1 pear.

Sugar-free Jell-O

¾ cup cottage cheese with: 1 tsp. honey or 1 tbsp. peanuts or 1 tbsp. berries or apple chunks

1 cup of almond milk with ½ cup blueberries.

5 celery sticks and 5 baby carrots with 2 tbsp. hummus and 3 dill pickles.

3 sliced radishes with a little salt and 5 cucumber slices and a wedge of Laughing Cow cream cheese.

Baked tortilla chips with salsa. You can also add some guacamole; here is a fast and delicious way to make it: take 1 avocado, scoop into a bowl and mash with a fork then add some Pico de Gallo and mix. Better if you can let stand for a short time for the flavors to blend.

Thin sliced provolone cheese and top with a slice of Canadian bacon then roll up; serve 2 rolls.

Sliced tomato with a drizzle of olive oil and a sprinkle of Feta cheese.

Easy side dishes include:

> *Creamy Cucumbers* – Mix ½ cup no-fat yogurt, dash of salt, dash of dill weed, a cup of sliced onion and 2 cups of thinly sliced cucumbers; cover and refrigerate about 4 hours.

> *Cucumbers and cream cheese dip* – for the dip combine 2 or 3 wedges of the Laughing Cow cream cheese (45 calories per wedge), chopped green onion and some dill then mix. Either spread on cucumber slices or dip them.

Broccoli slaw – this comes in a bag so you can mix your own dressing to add to it; a quick and easy dressing for your slaw is mix low-fat mayonnaise with sesame oil for an Asian slaw. Or mix a small amount of low-fat mayonnaise with Dijon mustard and some balsamic vinegar and toss with the slaw. Another option is to add some sliced pecans and/or dried cranberries, or diced apples.

Spicy Mushrooms – mix together ½ cup fat free Italian dressing, a teaspoon of crushed basil leaves and about 4 cups of sliced mushrooms. Serve cold by covering and refrigerate for 4 hours or serve hot by sautéing in a pan until mushrooms are soft.

Baked Tomato & Eggplant – take sliced tomatoes and thinly sliced eggplant; cook the eggplant in a skillet in a small amount of olive oil for a few minutes. Then in a baking dish layer the eggplant with tomato slices seasoning each layer with a little parsley, salt and pepper. Cover and bake for an hour.

Mashed butter beans – this is a great substitute for mashed potatoes; mash up cooked butter beans then mix with chicken broth and low-calorie butter.

Steamed Spinach – using a steamer lightly steam the spinach leaves then top with pepper, garlic, olive oil and a squeeze of lemon.

Sautéed New Potatoes – take a can of new potatoes, slice them in half and sauté in a pan with a small amount of olive oil, garlic (or garlic salt), salt

and pepper until they are lightly browned. Add
slices white onions while cooking for added flavor.
Potatoes are high on the glycemic index level so
keep portions very small.

Vegetables such as cauliflower, broccoli, and asparagus are
always a good choice as a side; steaming your vegetables is
a common method for preparation, but also try sautéing
them in small amount of olive oil with different spices. Even
broccoli and cauliflower can be cooked this way; it's simple
and a great variation to steaming. My favorite is to heat a
small amount of olive oil, about a teaspoon, sauté some
chopped green onion then toss in some fresh spinach leaves
and arugula and continue to sauté until the leaves start to
wilt which only takes a couple of minutes; add some salt
and pepper and you have a quick, tasty and healthy side.

Another way to cook vegetables is grilling them; simply
brush with olive oil and sprinkle with salt then grill. Most
tender vegetables if you slice lengthwise can go right on the
grill such as squash, zucchini, and eggplant. Even cabbage
can be grilled; cut a head of cabbage in quarters, brush with
olive oil and grill; then chop it up and drizzle with some
vinaigrette topped with gorgonzola or feta cheese. One
other option is to use skewers; thread cherry tomatoes,
sweet onion, and any other vegetable you choose on a
skewer. Coat with some olive oil, lemon juice and spices
such as rosemary and sea salt then grill. It's simple, healthy
and delicious.

Here are some recipes for appetizers and/or sides under 200 calories (most under 100):

Broccoli Soup

2 Servings

¾ cup chopped onion
2 tsp olive oil
¼ tsp tarragon
4 ½ cup broccoli florets
1 tbsp flour
1 cup water, divided
2 cup chicken broth
1 tsp white wine vinegar
½ tsp ground black pepper
1 tbsp shredded baby carrot

In a saucepan, mix onion, oil, tarragon, broccoli and a dash of salt. Stir over medium heat about 3 minutes. In a bowl, whisk flour and 2 tablespoons of the water until smooth then set aside.

In the saucepan, add broth, vinegar, pepper and remaining water; bring close to a boil then reduce heat and simmer about 10 minutes.

Puree soup mixture in a blender then return to the saucepan; whisk in flour mixture and stir over medium-high heat until it starts to thicken. Sprinkle with shredded carrot on top.

Thick and Creamy Low-fat Tomato Soup

8 Servings

1 tsp dried basil
2 tbsp olive oil
1 small onion finely chopped
1 ½ tsp dried oregano
6 cloves of garlic, minced or finely chopped
2 cups milk
2 cups chicken broth
2 cans crushed tomato
½ teaspoon salt and ground black pepper
1 tbsp balsamic vinegar

In a saucepan heat olive oil then add basil, onion and oregano and sauté. Add remaining ingredients of milk, garlic, chicken broth, crushed tomatoes, balsamic vinegar, salt and pepper then simmer for about 45 minutes.

Sprinkle with parmesan cheese and whole wheat croutons on top.

Spinach and Cheese Soup

8 Servings

8 oz fresh baby spinach leaves with stems removed
2 ½ cups milk (2% is best)
3 cups vegetable or chicken broth
1 cup low-fat cream cheese (Laughing Cow Swiss cheese)

In a large saucepan add spinach, milk and broth; bring to a boil then reduce heat and simmer for about 10-12 minutes. Remove from heat and let cool.

Once completely cool pour soup into a food processor or blender, chop the cheese into chunks and add to the soup then blend or process until smooth and creamy. Cover and chill in refrigerator for 3-4 hours before serving. Season with salt and pepper to taste.

Option: Sprinkle with parmesan cheese and whole wheat croutons on top.

Black Bean Soup

2 Servings

½ cup chopped onion
2 tsp olive oil
1 tsp minced garlic
¾ tsp cumin
¾ tsp oregano
1 can black beans, rinsed and drained
2 cup chicken broth
1 tbsp feta cheese

In a saucepan, mix onion, oil, garlic, cumin, oregano and a dash of salt; cook stirring constantly over medium heat about 3 minutes until softened. Stir in beans and broth, reduce heat and simmer stirring occasionally for about 10 minutes.

Serve with feta cheese sprinkled on top.

Sesame Hummus

4 Servings

1 can garbanzo beans, rinsed and drained
2 tbsp sesame seed
3 tbsp non-fat plain yogurt
2 tbsp water
2 tbsp lemon juice
1 tbsp low-sodium soy sauce
¼ tsp cumin
1 chopped green onion
1 garlic clove, minced

In a food processor combine beans and sesame seed then blend until smooth; add remaining ingredients and process until smooth then store in refrigerator.

Serve with assorted raw vegetables or pita bread.

Easy Guacamole

3-4 Servings

2 avocados
½ cup Pico de Gallo
½ tsp garlic salt
Squeeze of lime juice

Cut avocados in half, scoop out of skin with a large spoon and place in a bowl; mash with a fork then add the remaining ingredients and mix together. Let sit in refrigerator for about 20 minutes for flavors to blend.

Serve with assorted raw vegetables or baked tortilla chips.

Baked Kale

2 Servings

4 cups fresh kale
1 tbsp olive oil
Dash of salt and pepper

Preheat oven to 425 degrees. In a bowl toss kale with olive oil and season with salt and pepper. Spread kale in a single layer on a baking sheet then bake for about 6-8 minutes until crispy.

Broiled Spinach

4 Servings

1 pound fresh spinach leaves, stems removed
¼ tsp salt
Olive oil spray

Preheat broiler. On a sheet of heavy-duty foil spray with olive oil then place spinach on foil, sprinkle with salt and toss. Fold foil and seal edges to form a pouch; cook in broiler (or place on grill) for 8-10 minutes until leaves are wilted. Season with a dash of salt and pepper; top with sesame seeds as an option.

Creamed Spinach

4 Servings

1 package frozen chopped spinach (9 oz.)
1 tsp olive oil
2 tbsp chopped green onion
1/3 cup light sour cream
¼ cup skim milk
2 tbsp shredded mozzarella cheese
2 tsp flour
Dash of salt

Prepare the spinach as directed on the package; drain and dry by pressing with paper towels. Heat oil in large skillet over medium heat; add onion and sauté for about a minute.

Mix together the sour cream, milk, cheese, flour and salt then stir into the onions. Continue cooking until it thickens and is bubbly then stir the spinach into the sauce.

Broccoli-Carrot-Onion Slaw

2 Servings

¼ cup slivered baby carrots
½ cup chopped broccoli florets
¼ cup slivered red onion
1 tbsp light mayonnaise
1 tsp Dijon mustard

In a bowl, whisk the mayonnaise and mustard. Add broccoli, onion and carrots. Toss to coat.

Baked Cajun Cabbage in Cheese Sauce

4 Servings

1 head of cabbage
½ cup cold water (divided)
1 cup chopped onion
1 cup chopped celery
1 cup chopped green bell pepper
3 tbsp cornstarch
1 ½ cup skim milk
½ cup fat-free shredded cheddar cheese
Dash of cayenne pepper and salt
1 cup chopped green onion
¼ cup Italian bread crumbs

Remove outer leaves and heart from cabbage; cut into bite size sections and boil about 10 minutes until tender/crisp. Drain and set aside.

In a separate saucepan add ¼ cup water and sauté onion, celery and cayenne pepper for about 10 minutes. Add milk then stir in cornstarch and the remaining ¼ cup water; stir over medium-low heat until creamy then add cheese.

Place cabbage in casserole dish and top with cheese sauce; sprinkle with green onion and bread crumbs then bake at 350 degrees for about 30 minutes.

Mexican Cabbage

4 Servings

1 head of cabbage
1 can tomatoes and green chilies
1 thinly sliced onion
2 tbsp vinegar
Dash of salt

Place thinly sliced onions in bottom of casserole dish; chop cabbage and place over onions. Pour tomatoes and green chilies on top of cabbage and sprinkle with salt and vinegar.

Cover and bake for 20 minutes at 350 degrees for 25 minutes.

Spiced Mashed Sweet Potatoes

6 Servings

4 sweet potatoes
½ cup orange juice
2 tbsp brown sugar
2 tsp cinnamon
1 tsp chili powder
Dash of salt

Cook sweet potatoes either in oven or microwave until they are soft. While the potatoes cool mix in a bowl the rest of the ingredients.

Scoop the sweet potatoes out of the skins into a large bowl, add the orange juice mixture and mash well.

Cauliflower Mash

4 Servings

2 heads of cauliflower (washed and cut into chunks)
2 tbsp light butter
½ tsp sea salt

Cook/steam cauliflower until they are soft.

Then puree in a food processor or mash very well.

Reheat in pan; stir in salt and add pepper to taste.

Options: steam cauliflower with garlic; use half olive oil and half butter; add chives or chopped green onion.

Tomato Gazpacho

4 Servings

5 tomatoes
1 ½ cups cucumber, chopped
½ cup green onion, chopped
¼ cup red onion, chopped
1 garlic clove, minced
1 tsp seeded jalapeno, minced
1 tbsp vinegar
1 tbsp olive oil
Dash of salt

Cut up tomatoes and mix with the rest of the ingredients in a blender. Chill for about 30 minutes then serve with chopped avocado on top.

Lemon Cauliflower

4 Servings

2 cups cauliflower florets
1 tbsp butter, melted
1 tbsp drained capers, rinsed
1 tbsp lemon juice
1 ½ tsp each of chopped parsley and chives

Steam cauliflower until softened; while still hot add the remaining ingredients and mix.

Option: add red and green bell peppers to cauliflower.

Vegetables and Brown Rice

2 Servings

2 tsp olive oil
½ cup chopped green onions
1 small clove of garlic, minced
½ cup sliced mushrooms
½ cup sliced zucchini
¼ cup diced red bell pepper
1 tbsp soy sauce (low sodium)
1 cup cooked brown rice
Dash of pepper

Heat oil in a large skillet over medium heat; sauté onions and garlic until softened then add mushrooms, zucchini and red pepper and continue to sauté another 5 minutes.

Next add soy sauce and cooked rice with pepper and stir; continue to cook stirring often until heated through.

Herbed Rice Pilaf

4 Servings

3 tbsp minced red onion
1 ½ tbsp minced baby carrot
2 tsp canola oil
¾ tsp thyme
¾ cup instant brown rice
1 ¼ cup chicken broth

In a saucepan, combine onion, carrot, oil, thyme and salt to taste. Cook, stirring over medium heat until sizzling (about 2 minutes). Add rice, stir to coat with seasonings. Add broth, bring to a boil. Reduce heat and cover so mixture simmers for 12 minutes.

Remove from heat and let sit for 5 minutes; fluff with fork.

Sautéed Greek Kale

4 Servings

2 tbsp chopped red onion
2 tsp olive oil
¼ tsp oregano
1 ½ cup packed chopped kale leaves
2 tsp feta cheese
Pinch of red pepper flakes

In a skillet, combine onion, oil, oregano and salt to taste. Cook over medium heat, stirring until softened, about 3 minutes. Add kale and stir to coat. Cover and cook for 2 minutes stirring occasionally. Stir in red pepper flakes.

Sprinkle with crumbled feta and serve.

Pureed Black Beans

2 Servings

¼ cup minced red onion
2 tsp olive oil
1 tsp thyme
¼ tsp ground black pepper
1 cup canned black beans, rinsed and drained
½ cup chicken broth
1 tsp lemon juice
½ tsp grated lemon peel

Heat oil in a large skillet over medium heat; sauté onions and garlic until softened then add mushrooms, zucchini and red pepper and continue to sauté another 5 minutes.

Next add soy sauce and cooked rice with pepper and stir; continue to cook stirring often until heated through.

French Carrots

2 Servings

1 ¼ cup baby carrots
2 tsp butter
1 tbsp minced red onion
¼ tsp tarragon
¼ cup chicken broth
1 tbsp light sour cream
1 tsp minced parsley

Combine carrots, butter, onion, tarragon in a saucepan with salt, cook over medium heat, stirring, about 3 minutes. Add broth, cover and reduce heat to simmer about 10 minutes. Stir in sour cream, serve sprinkle with parsley.

Sweet & Sour Broccoli

2 Servings

2 tbsp minced red onion
2 tsp olive oil
1 tsp minced garlic
½ tsp oregano
1 ¾ cup broccoli florets, chopped
½ cup canned diced tomatoes, with juice
1 tbsp raisins

In a skillet, combine onion, oil, garlic, oregano; cook over low heat about 2 minutes. Add broccoli and stir; cook until sizzling about another minute. Add tomatoes and raisins; cook until broccoli is crisp but tender, about 2 minutes.

Garlicky Chinese Broccoli

2 Servings

1 tbsp minced baby carrot
1 tbsp minced red onion
2 tsp canola oil
1 tsp minced garlic
1 tsp grated fresh ginger
1 bag (8 oz) broccoli florets, chopped
1 tbsp hot water

In a skillet combine carrot, onion, oil, garlic, ginger and dash of salt; cook over low heat for 3 minutes.

Add broccoli, stir to coat; add water and cover. Cook for 1 to 2 minutes stirring occasionally.

Desserts

There isn't a large section on dessert because while losing weight you want to avoid sugar which means you want to avoid desserts. But when an occasion calls for dessert fruit is a good option, keep it simple such as broiling with some cinnamon and/or honey. Try serving with some light whipped cream or with yogurt and honey.

Or try:

Chocolate covered fruit: melt about 2 tablespoons of semisweet chocolate chips then pour over sliced bananas and strawberries.

Fruit sorbet or light (low sugar) ice cream / frozen yogurt.

Frozen Hot Chocolate: combine ½ cup chocolate syrup, 1 cup fat-free evaporated milk, ½ tsp. vanilla extract, and 3 cups ice cube in a blender until smooth. Pour into cocktail glasses and top with a little low-fat whipped topping and some chocolate shavings.

Faux Apple Pie: mix chopped apple with some chopped walnuts and maple syrup.

Fruit Salad: in a large bowl add ½ bag of frozen pitted cherries and let defrost so that it creates a syrup; then add chopped apple, pear, peach, sliced strawberries and some fresh blueberries; mash up some fresh mint leaves and add to fruit then stir. You can eat right away but it's better if you let it sit a while in the refrigerator.

Chocolate Honey Bananas: melt a small amount of butter in a skillet, add about 4 bananas cut lengthwise in half and cook, turning occasionally for about 4 minutes. Arrange on 4 plates, drizzle with honey and sprinkle grated chocolate over each.

Pound cake with fruit: in a bowl add your choice of frozen fruit such as strawberries, blueberries, peaches and let thaw so that a juice is created. Pour over a loaf of pound cake; serve with some light whipped cream.

Cinnamon Baked Apples: mix together a tablespoon of butter, tablespoon of brown sugar and ¼ teaspoon of cinnamon; top apple slices or fill in a cored apple then bake for 30 to 40 minutes. Top with a small scoop of vanilla ice cream.

Chapter 9: Maintenance

The tips and recipes in this book are not just for losing weight; once you've reached your goal you can't go back to eating the way you used to. This is the way you will eat for life...for a long healthy life. When you are working on losing weight you will need to be a little stricter on the number of calories you take in each day. When losing weight your daily calorie intake depends on your height and amount of activity but on average it is about 1200-1600 calories a day; then once the weight is lost you can bump that up to about 1600-2000 a day again depending on the amount of activity.

You can bring some of your favorite foods back but control your portions. If you love steak, mashed potatoes or macaroni and cheese it doesn't mean you can never enjoy them again...you can on occasion or when you are at an event enjoy some of your favorite foods but in small portions. Have a few bites and eat them slowly and enjoy them; if you have ever seen a thin person eating some pasta and you wonder how they can do that the secret is enjoying just a small amount. To give you an idea of what a portion size is for pasta its ½ cup (cooked) which is about the size of an ice-cream scoop; then bulk it up with vegetables and lean protein.

So accept in your mind that you are going to eat healthy and exercise for life; remind yourself often how good it feels to eat healthy and exercise. Enjoy some of your favorite foods but do so with small portions. You will stop eating before you feel full then give your stomach time to catch up and avoid overeating. You will not eat when you are bored or stressed but will find other ways to take care of those emotions without food such as a hobby, exercise, meditation.

Always remember, it's just food, fuel for your body and you are in control of what you eat! But also have fun with food, if you have a craving for something...let's say a hamburger, come up with creative ways to satisfy that craving but keep it healthy. Try new foods, like a fruit or vegetable you have never eaten before; have you ever had plantain, bok choy, Swiss chard, starfruit or papaya? Come up with your own creative ways to eat healthy, experiment with healthy foods and make it fun.

Continue to eat whole, natural foods as much as possible. Maintain a healthy low-GI diet 85-90% of the time; studies show following a low-GI (glycemic-index) diet may give you the best chance of keeping the weight off in a healthy way. A low-GI diet is similar to a Mediterranean-style diet that emphasizes foods with slow digesting carbohydrates, such as beans and lentils, non-starchy vegetables, fruit and whole grains, plus lean proteins and healthy fats.

Continue with your food journal so if the weight comes creeping back on you can look at what you've been consuming. And note in your journal the reasons why you want to stay slim and healthy, remind yourself how good you feel and how you have more energy.

Over time it will become routine, second nature, to follow a healthy lifestyle. Remember to eat until you are satisfied, not until you are full. But also don't let yourself get too hungry, then you run the risk of overeating. Plan on what you can have as a small snack for mid-morning and mid-afternoon to prevent yourself from getting too hungry. Something simple like a handful of almonds, fruit, a healthy snack bar, etc.; just keep it around 100-150 calories.

Two words to remember for maintaining a healthy weight...balance and moderation. Eat the right balance of protein, carbs and fat. And eat what you love in moderation.

Chapter 10: Eating Out

The key to losing weight and eating healthy is to prepare your own meals so you know what you are eating; but we can't give up on eating out completely. It's become a little easier with many restaurants and fast-food chains offering healthier options and making nutritional content available to help you make better choices. But you still need to beware of meals when eating out that sound healthy but are not.

Most restaurant chains provide the nutritional information on their website, so if you know what restaurant you are going to look at their website before and decide what you will eat.

If it is a restaurant that does not provide the nutritional information then be sure to read what is included in the meal and know what you are getting. Chicken and fish always seem like a healthy choice but beware of sauces served with it or if it is breaded and fried then it's not a good choice.

For example at Chili's you may think the Boneless Buffalo Chicken Salad sounds like a healthy selection but the chicken is breaded and fried, there is bacon and the Pico de Gallo-ranch dressing is full of calories and fat; this salad has 920 calories! Or at Olive Garden the Chicken and Shrimp Carbonara sounds healthy, after all it has chicken and shrimp right? But the flavor and the fat are in the white cream sauce bringing the calorie count on this dish up to 1440 calories. That's almost a full days' worth of calories in one dish. And there is the Cajun Shrimp & Chicken Pasta at T.G.I. Friday's and you think shrimp and chicken are both low fat options but add in the butter and the cream and cheese, you are looking at 1010 calories!

Here are a few more examples of chicken dishes to avoid and better options:

Chicken Quesadilla at Baja Fresh has 1330 calories and the veggie quesadilla has 1260 because the large flour tortilla, the cheese, guacamole and sour cream. A better option would be 2 tacos.

Grilled Chicken and Avocado Club at Cheesecake Factory is a whopping 1752 calories; in fact most of the sandwiches on the menu there are high in calories. Stick to their new SkinnyLicous menu which will also help narrow down the time you would normally spend going through their pages of menu selections.

At Panda Express everyone loves the Orange Chicken which alone is 420 calories, that doesn't sound too bad however the calories from fat are 180 which is the highest of the chicken entrees. Plus if you add steamed rice at 380 calories you can see that adding up. A better choice is the Sweet & Sour Chicken Breast at 380 although the calories from fat are still high at 150. So an even better choice is the Black Pepper Chicken or Mushroom Chicken with Mixed Veggies as a side instead of rice.

The California Chicken Sandwich at Red Robin sounds like a better option to their hamburgers but it's at 744 calories due to the mayo, the bacon and guacamole. The Keep It Simple burger is actually a better choice with 569 calories.

These are all chain restaurants so you can look this information up and determine the bad choices but when eating where you do not have the calories available just remember to consider how it is cooked, what it is cooked in and what is included with it.

Avoid anything fried, avoid butter, mayonnaise, cream sauces, dressings and heavy cheese. And watch your portion sizes; when it comes to food...size does matter. Consider splitting a meal which will save money and calories; or save half to take home for the next meal. You could also order an appetizer as your meal or a small salad and small appetizer.

Also avoid buffets or all-you-can-eat specials but if it's not up to you then use the small plate such as a salad plate and choose lots of vegetable; then eat slowly and enjoy so you won't be tempted to overeat.

Again if you are going to a chain restaurant then the nutritional information is available on their website so use it! Many fast-food chains have added healthy menu items so if you can't bring your lunch to work or need to pick up something fast there are some good alternatives.

 Here are some examples of what is currently on the menus at popular fast-food restaurants:

McDonalds

Hamburger: 250 calories / 9 grams fat   (suggested meal is with apple slices or side salad)

Chicken McNuggets (6): 280 calories / 18 grams fat (does not include calories for dipping sauce)

Premium Grilled Chicken Sandwich: 350 calories / 9 grams fat

Premium Caesar Salad w/ Caesar dressing: 380 calories / 24 grams fat

Apple Slices: 15 calories / no fat

Side Salad: 20 calories / no fat

Newman's Own Low Fat Balsamic Vinaigrette: 35 calories / 2.5 grams fat

Fruit & Walnuts: 210 calories / 8 grams fat

Vanilla Reduced Fat Ice Cream Cone: 170 calories / 4.5 grams fat

Egg McMuffin: 300 calories / 12 grams fat

Fruit & Maple Oatmeal: 290 calories / 4.5 grams fat

Bad Choices: Quarter w/ Cheese is 520 calories / Angus Delux is 750 calories / Premium Grilled Chicken Club Sandwich is 460 calories / McRib is 500 calories / Chicken Selects Premium Breast Strips (5pc) is 640 calories / Small French Fries is 230 calories / Big Breakfast (large with biscuit) is 800 calories (Regular size is 740 calories)

Keep in mind if ordering a coffee drinks, those have as many calories as a meal. A Medium Non-Fat Caramel Mocha is a better choice but still has 240 calories; so choose this as a mid-morning snack if you want but not with your meal. If you got to McDonalds website and look up the nutritional information there are several pages of just the drinks and the coffee drinks depending on the size, if it's non-fat or sugar-free so do your homework.

Burger King

Whopper Jr: 340 calories / 18 grams fat (compared to a Whopper at 670 calories)

Whopper Jr w/o Mayo: 260 calories / 9 grams fat (good choice with apple slices as a side)

Hamburger: 240 calories / 8 grams fat

Tendergrill Chicken Sandwich: 470 calories / 18 grams fat

Tendergrill Chicken Sandwich w/o Mayo: 360 calories / 6 grams fat

Chicken Nuggets (6): 290 calories / 17 grams fat

Veggie Burger: 410 calories / 16 grams fat

Veggie Burger w/o Mayo: 320 calories / 7 grams fat

Garden Fresh Salad Chicken, Apple & Cranberry with Tendergrill and dressing: 520 calories / 26 grams fat

Breakfast Muffin Sandwich, Egg & Cheese: 220 calories / 9 grams fat

Oatmeal Original: 140 calories / 3.5 grams fat

Bad Choices: Whopper is 670 calories and 40 grams fat / Original Chicken Sandwich is 630 calories and 39 grams fat / Garden Fresh Salad Chicken Caesar with Tendercrisp and dressing is 670 calories and 43 grams fat / Ultimate Breakfast Platter is 1450 calories and 84 grams fat

Carl's Jr.

Trim It Famous Star: 430 calories / 17 grams fat

Charbroiled BBQ Chicken Sandwich: 380 calories / 7 grams fat

The Low Carb Charbroiled BBQ Chicken Sandwich: 180 calories / 4.5 grams fat

Kid's Hamburger: 280 calories / 10 grams fat

Chicken Stars (6): 260 calories / 16 grams fat

Original Grilled Chicken Salad: 280 calories / 13 grams fat

Cranberry Apple Walnut Chicken Salad: 330 calories / 15 grams fat

Low Fat Balsamic Vinaigrette Dressing: 35 calories / 1.5 grams fat

Bad Choices: Famous Star with Cheese is 680 calories / Super Star with Cheese is 940 calories / Turkey Burger is 490 calories / Charbroiled Santa Fe Chicken Sandwich is 570 calories / Small Natural Cut Fries are 310 calories / Steak & Egg Burrito is 640 calories / Loaded Breakfast Burrito is 780 calories

Wendy's

Jr. Hamburger: 250 calories / 10 grams fat

Grilled Chicken Go Wrap: 260 calories / 10 grams fat

Ultimate Chicken Grill Sandwich: 390 calories / 10 grams fat

Apple Pecan Chicken Salad: 350 calories / 11 grams fat

BLT Cobb Salad: 390 calories / 20 grams fat

Caesar Side Salad: 60 calories / 3.5 grams fat

Lemon Garlic Caesar Dressing: 110 calories / 11 grams fat

Garden Side Salad: 25 calories / no fat

Light Classic Ranch Dressing: 50 calories / 4.5 grams fat

Plain Baked Potato: 270 calories / no fat

Sour Cream & Chives Baked Potato: 320 calories / 3.5 grams fat

Small Chili: 210 calories / 6 grams fat

5 pc Chicken Nuggets: 220 calories / 14 grams fat

Bad Choices: ¼ Pound Single Burger is 580 calories / Baconater is 970 calories / Homestyle Chicken Filet Sandwich is 560 calories / Asiago Ranch Club w/ Homestyle Chicken is 730 calories / Baja Salad is 540 calories / Medium Natural Cut Fries are 420 calories / Small Chocolate Frosty is 300 calories

Subway

6" Black Forest Ham: 290 calories / 4.5 grams fat

6" Subway Club: 310 calories / 4.5 grams fat

6" Turkey Breast: 280 calories / 3.5 grams fat

6" Veggie Delight: 230 calories / 2.5 grams fat

*these are based on 9-grain wheat bread, lettuce, tomatoes, onions, green peppers and cucumbers.

Double Chicken Chopped Salad: 220 calories / 4.5 grams fat

Subway Club Salad: 140 calories / 3.5 grams fat

Turkey Breast and Ham Salad: 110 calories / 2.5 grams fat

*Salads do not include dressing; best choices for dressings are Fat Free Italian at 35 calories or Honey Mustard at 80 calories.

Roasted Chicken Noodle Soup: 110 calories / 2 grams fat

Tomato Garden Vegetable w/ Rotini Soup: 90 calories / 0 grams fat

Egg White & Cheese Muffin Melt: 150 calories / 3.5 grams fat

Egg White & Cheese on 3" Flatbread: 170 calories / 5 grams fat

6" Omelet Sandwich (egg white): 320 calories / 8 grams fat

Sides: sides are not needed, we have trained our minds that we need a side but a 6" sandwich is a complete meal; if you need a side then apple slices are the best choice at 35 calories or Baked Lays at 130 calories and eat only half the bag and save the rest for another meal.

Bad Choices: 6" Philly Cheesesteak is 500 calories / 6" Tuna is 470 calories / 6" Meatball Marinara is 480 calories / 6" Mega Melt Omelet Sandwich is 550 calories or on Flatbread is 620 calories

Taco Bell (stick to the Fresco Menu)

Fresco Bean Burrito: 350 calories / 9 grams fat

Fresco Burrito Supreme (Chicken): 340 calories / 8 grams fat

Fresco Chicken Soft Taco: 150 calories / 3.5 grams fat

Fresco Crunchy Taco: 140 calories / 8 grams fat

Fresco Grilled Steak Soft Taco: 150 calories / 4 grams fat

Chicken Soft Taco: 170 calories / 6 grams fat

Bean Burrito: 370 calories / 11 grams fat

Gordita Supreme – Chicken or Steak: 270 calories / 10 or 11 grams fat

Sausage and Egg Burrito: 270 calories / 15 grams fat

Bad Choices: Burrito Supreme-Beef is 420 calories / XXL Grilled Stuft Burrito – Beef is 880 calories / Nachos BellGrande is 760 calories / Fiesta Taco Salad – Chicken is 720 calories / Cantina Bowl is 560 calories / Chicken Quesadilla is 520 calories

Arby's

Roast Beef Classic: 350 calories / 12 grams fat

Jr. Roast Beef: 20 calories / 6 grams fat

Jr. Ham & Cheddar Melt: 210 calories / 6 grams fat

Jr. Chicken Sandwich: 320 calories / 15 grams fat

Turkey Classic: 290 calories / 5 grams fat

Chopped Farmhouse Salad – Roast Turkey: 240 calories / 13 grams fat (without dressing)

Light Italian Dressing: 20 calories / 1 gram fat

Side: Apple Slices at 35 calories (avoid the fries and potato cakes)

Bad Choices (pretty much everything else): Beef 'n Cheddar Classic is 440 calories / 'Shroom & Swiss is 510 calories / Roast Turkey, Ranch & Bacon Market Fresh Sandwich is 800 calories / Chicken Bacon & Swiss – Crispy is 610 calories / Prime-Cut Chicken Tenders (5) is 590 calories w/o sauce / Small Curly Fries are 400 calories / Potato Cakes (2) are 230 calories

KFC

Original Chicken Breast w/o skin: 160 calories / 3.5 grams fat

Original Chicken Whole Wing or Drumstick: 120 calories / 7 grams fat

Grilled Chicken Breast: 220 calories / 7 grams fat

Grilled Drumstick: 90 calories / 4 grams fat

KFC Original Filet: 200 calories / 9 grams fat

Original Recipe Bites (6): 200 calories / 9 grams fat

Chicken Little Sandwich w/o Sauce: 230 calories / 8 grams fat

Honey BBQ Sandwich: 320 calories / 3.5 grams fat

Grilled Drumstick Value Box: 380 calories / 19 grams fat

Sides:

House Side Salad: 15 calories / no fat

Light Italian Dressing: 15 calories / .5 grams fat

Fat-Free Ranch Dressing: 35 calories / no fat (compared to regular Ranch at 160 calories / 17 grams fat)

Green Beans: 25 calories / no fat

Mashed Potatoes w/o Gravy: 90 calories / 3 grams fat

Corn on the Cob (3"): 70 calories / .5 grams fat (no butter)

Bad Choices: Original Chicken Breast with Skin is 360 calories / Popcorn Chicken is 400 calories or 560 calories for the large / Crispy Twister Sandwich is 610 calories / Chicken Pot Pie is 790 calories / KFC Famous Bowl – Mashed Potato with Gravy is 680 calories / Potato wedges are 290 calories / Potato Salad is 210 calories / 1 Biscuit is 180 calories

Boston Market

Quarter White Rotisserie Chicken Meal (no skin) with Garlic Dill New Potatoes and Fresh Steamed Vegetables: 410 calories / 2 grams fat

Roasted Turkey Breast Meal (regular) with Fresh Vegetable Stuffing and Fresh Steamed Vegetables: 480 calories / 18 grams fat

Meals under 550 Calories include:

Quarter White Chicken Meal (skinless) with Garlicky Spinach and Fresh Steamed Vegetables is 420 calories / with Garlic Dill Potatoes and Fresh Steamed Vegetables is 400 calories / with Sweet Corn and Garlic Dill Potatoes is 440 calories

Turkey Regular with Garlicky Spinach and Garlic Dill Potatoes is 400 calories / with Garlicky Spinach and Stuffing is 520 calories / with Mashed Potatoes and Fresh Steamed Vegetables is 500 calories

Bad Choices: most of the meals are high in calories and fat during weight loss; stick to the Skinless White Rotisserie Chicken with Steamed Vegetables.

Panda Express

Mushroom Chicken: 180 calories / 9 grams fat

String Bean Chicken Breast: 160 calories / 6 grams fat

Broccoli Beef: 120 calories / 4 grams fat

Peppercorn Shrimp: 170 calories / 5 grams fat

Served with:

Mixed Veggies (side): 70 calories / .5 grams fat

Veggie Spring Roll: 160 calories / 7 grams fat

Chicken Egg Roll: 200 calories / 12 grams fat

Bad Choices: Chow Mein is 490 calories / Fried Rice is 530 calories / Steamed Rice is 380 calories / Orange Chicken is 420 calories / Beijing Beef is 690 calories / Honey Walnut Shrimp is 370 calories

Starbucks
Drinks (Grande with 2% Milk):

Caffe Latte: 190 calories / 7 grams fat

Iced Caffe Latte: 130 calories / 4.5 grams fat

Cappuccino: 120 calories / 4 grams fat

Skinny Caramel Macchiato: 140 calories / 1 gram fat

Skinny Cinnamon Dolce Latte: 180 calories / 6 grams fat

Tazo Shaken Iced Green Tea Lemonade (unsweetened): 45 calories / no fat (*sweetened is 130 calories)

Tall Iced Skinny Latte: 60 calories / no fat

Tall Nonfat Tazo Green Tea Latte: 150 calories / no fat

Tall Skinny Vanilla Latte: 90 calories / no fat

Bad Choices (Grande): Caffe Mocha is 260 calories / Peppermint White Chocolate Mocha is 440 calories / White Chocolate Mocha is 400 calories / Cinnamon Dolce Frappuccino Blended Beverage is 350 calories / Tazo Green Tea Latte (sweetened) is 350 calories

Food:

Everything with Cheese Bagel: 280 calories / 2 grams fat

Multigrain Bagel: 300 calories / 3 grams fat

Plain Bagel: 280 calories / 1 gram fat

*Petite Vanilla Bean Scone: 140 calories / 5 grams fat

*Marshmallow Dream Bar: 210 calories / 4 grams fat

*Reduced-fat Very Berry Coffee Cake: 350 calories / 10 grams fat

*Reduced-fat Cinnamon Swirl Coffee Cake: 340 calories / 9 grams fat

　　　*Beware of high sugar content

Chicken & Hummus Bistro Box: 260 calories / 7 grams fat

Goat Cheese & Garden Veggies Bistro Box: 220 calories / 10 grams fat

Ham & Swiss Panini: 340 calories / 10 grams fat

Roasted Vegetable Panini: 350 calories / 12 grams fat

Turkey & Swiss Sandwich: 390 calories / 13 grams fat

Spinach & Feta Breakfast Wrap: 290 calories / 10 grams fat

Perfect Oatmeal: 140 calories / 2.5 grams fat

Turkey Bacon & White Cheddar Breakfast Sandwich: 320 calories / 7 grams fat

Greek Yogurt with Honey Parfait: 300 calories / 12 grams fat

Peach Raspberry Yogurt Parfait: 280 calories / 3.5 grams fat

Strawberry Blueberry Yogurt Parfait: 290 calories / 3.5 grams fat

Bad Choices: Banana Nut Loaf is 490 calories / Blueberry Scone is 460 calories / Cheese Danish is 420 calories / Iced Lemon Pound Cake is 490 calories / Zucchini Walnut Muffin is 490 calories / Sausage & Cheddar Classic Breakfast Sandwich is 500 calories / Egg Salad Sandwich is 460 calories

Remember: meals over 400 calories are not good choices when losing weight but acceptable when maintaining. Also keep in mind that menus change so check the websites to confirm the nutritional information.

Homework:

Trying to remember this nutritional information is impossible; so to help you when you need to pick up lunch or dinner you have some homework to do. Make a list like the one shown as an example with some of the fast-food and/or restaurants near your home or work where you will usually stop to pick up lunch or dinner. Then go to their websites and choose 3 meals that you like and add up to 400 calories or less and write them in on your list. Keep this list with you, or make copies and keep one at work, in your car, etc. By keeping your choices limited there is less room for error.

For example, if you list McDonalds you could put down as one of your meal selections a Hamburger at 250 calories with a side salad and low-fat balsamic dressing at 55 calories for a total of 305 calories.

A second choice could be a hamburger at 250 calories and a small vanilla cone at 170 calories which is 420 calories so that's pushing the maximum on calories and sugar but ok once in a while. And a third choice could be a Grilled Chicken Sandwich at 350 calories with apple slices at 15 for a total of 365 calories.

If you want to include a drink include the calories for that drink but stick to water as much as possible because we know the benefits of water and you don't have to add calories for it. Occasionally have a diet drink keeping in mind you want to keep the artificial sweeteners to a minimum.

Consider completing one for lunch/dinner and another list for breakfast.

Name of Restaurant/Fast Food

_____

Meal Choices:

1. _____

   _____ = _____Calories

2. _____

   _____ = _____Calories

3. _____

   _____ = _____Calories

Name of Restaurant/Fast Food

_____

Meal Choices:

1. _____

   _____ = _____Calories

2. _____

   _____ = _____Calories

3. _____

   _____ = _____Calories

For restaurants that are not chains and do not provide nutritional information follow these guidelines:

Mexican Restaurants

There are a lot of calories in Mexican food with the cheese and more cheese, guacamole, sour cream, flour tortillas, refried beans and usually large portions. When dining out at a Mexican restaurant the best choices are chicken fajitas or tacos with grilled chicken or fish. Corn tortillas are better than flour and try to limit how much tortilla you eat. When eating tacos to save some calories you can eat them with a fork and eat the meat, lettuce, tomato with only a little cheese and little tortilla and you can add a small amount of guacamole and/or sour cream. Also choose black beans over refried beans and avoid the rice. You will still enjoy the meal and feel better about the choices you made. Also limit the chips and salsa before the meal, the salsa isn't bad but the chips will add up. And avoid the margarita unless it's a skinny type or go with a light beer.

Italian Restaurants

When eating Italian stay away from the cream sauces! A red marinara sauce is a better choice or a light olive oil or pesto sauce. Avoid a lot of cheese, so although lasagna has a red sauce it also has a lot of cheese and fatty beef or sausage so be wary. Go with a light pasta with lean meat and veggies; pasta primavera is a good choice. And skip the bread unless they offer some wheat types of bread but remember you are taking in a lot of carbs with the pasta. Go with a broth based soup or salad with a vinaigrette dressing before the meal and keep your pasta portion small.

And when eating out keep these tips in mind:

Prepare before you go; if possible check out the menu before and determine what your best choices are.

Be mindful of what you are eating and how much. When eating out with friends it's easy to start chatting and not think about what you are eating which can lead to overeating. The plus side to eating out with friends is you are chatting and eating slower but pay attention to what you are eating and how much.

Order water and if having alcohol limit your intake and sip your water in between sipping your drink; stick to wine, light beer or if having a cocktail avoid sugary mixers.

Avoid snacking too much on the pre-meal freebies or appetizers (unless you are having an appetizer as your meal).

Feel free to ask for modifications such as if ordering a sandwich that comes with mayo ask for mustard instead; if it comes with a baked potato ask for the butter on the side.

Watch your portions; possibly share the meal with a friend or if it's a large portion divide it up and take half home then have it for breakfast.

And if you are going to indulge stick to the 3-bite rule; enjoy 3 bites then you are done.

Summary

Make up your mind to change your life, to live a more healthy and active lifestyle. There is so much more in life to enjoy than food, food should not be a passion. Don't be afraid to talk about it, to ask for help if needed.

Points to remember are (yes we are going to hammer in these points again to help you remember):

Portion Control! Portion Control! Portion Control! The number one point to remember is to be mindful of the size of your portions; enjoy the foods you love in small portions is the key to keeping your weight in check.

Strive to eat whole, natural foods as much as possible. Load up on vegetables and fruit, include plant-based proteins such as nuts and legumes, use whole grains in moderation instead of refined carbohydrates, and select lean high quality meat and fish.

Eat 3 regular meals with 2 snacks in between or try eating 5 small meals a day to keep the metabolic fire burning. Plan your snacks or small meals for the day so you can take them to work.

Eat slowly and calmly to allow your digestive system to function properly. Enjoy your meals!

When you are full, stop eating! You do not need to clean your plate; it's ok to leave some food on your plate.

And don't eat mindlessly such as when eating something that tastes so good you want to keep eating more but take control and stop. Remind yourself its only food, it does not have power over you, you have the power.

Eat breakfast every morning, one made up of protein and fiber (not sugar); it's one of the best things you can do to jump start your metabolism by bringing your blood sugar back to normal and help it stay steady through the day.

Eat only when you're hungry; beware of eating when you are bored.

Eat fruit instead of drinking it; fruit juice is typically loaded with sugar; real fruit will fill you up with less calories.

Drink lots of water but avoid the sugar-added flavored waters; if you need flavor add chunks of fruit. Also drink green tea daily and less coffee.

Exercise! Try to fit in a small amount daily with walks, biking, playing with your kids or dog; then have a strength training workout with some cardio 3 to 4 times a week. Especially as we age we lose muscle mass so exercise is crucial.

Your body needs to restore itself so get 7 to 8 hours of sleep every night to allow it to heal from the stress of the day. Not enough sleep has been linked to increased output of the hunger hormone, ghrelin, which leads to eating more.

When you feel weak focus on your goals and how good it feels when you lose a few pounds, how good you feel when you eat right and after you exercise; think about those feelings and find your strength.

Again what we talk about in this book is not a temporary change or fix but a change you are making to how you eat and exercise for life.

And every couple of months or so come back and read through this again, you will find some things you forgot and it will help get you back on track.

This is now your lifestyle basics:

1. Portion control
2. Avoid processed foods and stick to lean meat, vegetables and fruit as much as possible.
3. Drink lots of water!
4. Get 30-45 minutes of exercise at least 3 times a week, 5 times if possible.
5. Get plenty of sleep.
6. Get into a routine.

You have the power to set yourself up for success; look at each day as an opportunity to make smart choices that will improve your life now and for the future.

Directory of Vitamins and Supplements

Acai Berry - Acai berry is a powerful antioxidant fruit; it provides antioxidants that fight off and kill 'free radical molecules in our body. As a powerful antioxidant it may help boost weight loss but don't fall for the hype that this is a miracle fruit.

Apple Cider Vinegar - apple cider vinegar comes from pulverized apples and is touted as having many health benefits; for weight loss it is said to help you feel full and satisfied quicker but needs further research. Using it in a dressing is fine but because it is highly acidic there are risks to taking it in pure form or in pills such as it could cause damage to tooth enamel, it can cause low potassium and bone density.

Arginine – also known as L-Arginine is an amino acid produced in the body and found in many foods—especially those rich in protein, such as dairy products, meats, fish, nuts, and soybeans. Most of the time, we produce or consume all the arginine we need. There is no evidence that it works as a muscle builder.

B-12 – Vitamin B-12 is a water-soluble B complex vitamin found naturally in a variety of foods, including meat, fish and dairy products. It is offered at some clinics as a shot as part of a weight-loss program stating it provides more energy and boosts your metabolism; but unless you have a vitamin B-12 deficiency injections aren't likely to boost your energy or metabolism.

Calcium – taking calcium supplements boosts weight loss, but according to studies only in people whose diets are calcium deficient. Calcium is important for strong bones and important to other functions of the human body.

Chromium – Chromium picolinate is promoted as a nutritional supplement that works to increase the efficiency of insulin to optimal levels; the exact mechanisms by which chromium improves this insulin efficiency are currently unclear and further research is being done.

Coconut Water – it is fairly low in calories and is a good source of B vitamins and potassium. Coconut water also contains electrolytes, some plant hormones, enzymes, and amino acids so it could have some antioxidant benefits however it has not been well studied so there is little evidence of the benefits at this time.

Coenzyme Q10 – is a nutrient that occurs naturally in the body and is found in many foods we eat such as beef, soybeans and peanuts. It acts as an antioxidant which protects cells from damage and helps maintain heart health. It also protects muscles as an anti-inflammatory.

Creatine – is formed from amino acids and plays a role in converting food into energy; we get creatine naturally from meat and fish. It may boost stamina for sports and aerobic activity and it may increase muscle mass. But despite the wide use of creatine by athletes there is not much evidence to prove that.

DHEA – is a hormone that is naturally produced by the adrenal glands and decreases with age. Supplements may help with muscle strength and slow aging process but results from studies are unclear of this and there are possible side effects because this is a hormone such as headaches, sleep issues and more serious effects such as increased risk of heart problems and some cancers.

Fiber – is filling and has very few calories therefore high-fiber foods may help with weight loss; it can also slow the absorption of carbohydrates, helping to improve blood sugar levels. Fiber is found in whole foods such as a variety of fruits, vegetables, and grains.

Flaxseed – is a good source of fiber, antioxidants, and Omega-3 fatty plus vitamins such as B, magnesium, and manganese; but it is low in fat and carbohydrates. Try sprinkling some ground flaxseed in your cereal, oatmeal, soups, salads, etc.

Ginseng – is an herb used to improve both mental and physical health; it is also reported to increase energy and endurance, reduce fatigue and the effects of stress, and prevent infections.

Glucosamine – is a compound found naturally in the body to help with joints and repair of cartilage; the supplement is promoted as helping with mobility and flexibility.

Glucomannan – is derived from an Asian plant and is a fiber considered to help with blood sugar control; and since it is a fiber it may also help with suppressing appetite.

Grape Seed Extract – is known as being beneficial for a number of cardiovascular conditions and may help with poor circulation and high cholesterol. Grape seed extract also reduces swelling caused by injury and it contains antioxidants that protect cells from damage.

Guarana – is a stimulant containing caffeine said to increase mental alertness, fight fatigue, and increase stamina; it has become popular in energy drinks and teas. Like other stimulants Guarana can have serious side effects so use caution.

Kefir – is a probiotic with good bacteria and yeast to help balance your digestive system; it's like a liquid yogurt. It offers weight loss benefits by helping to maintain a healthy bowel functions and provides calcium for fat burning.

Magnesium – is a mineral necessary in the chemical reaction that allows insulin to move glucose into cells, where glucose is involved in making energy for the body; it also helps the body digest, absorb, and utilize proteins, fats, and carbohydrates. It is better to get your magnesium through food as it is more easily absorbed that way. Foods rich in magnesium include almonds, cashews, Brazil nuts, pumpkin seeds and whole grains but if you are not able to get an adequate amount then there are supplements.

Niacin – is also known as vitamin B3 and as part of the vitamin B complex helps regulate metabolism. Niacin though has an indirect effect on weight loss; it is an important nutrient but too much can have adverse effects and could even cause weight gain. It is found naturally in legumes, meats, fish, peanut butter and whole grains.

Omega-3 Fatty Acids – are found in found in deep-sea fish such as salmon, mackerel, and swordfish as well as certain oils and nuts. Research on the benefits of Omega-3 is ongoing but they might increase satiety, which decreases calorie intake. And there are health benefits such as lower blood pressure, lower triglycerides and reduces the risk of heart attack and stroke.

Potassium – is an essential dietary mineral and electrolyte which is stored inside our body cells and helps build muscle, balance electrolytes and aid the heart and kidneys to function properly. Potassium is lost in sweat so the more exercise the more you need to replenish it. We get potassium from potatoes with the skin and fruits such as bananas, plums, orange juice; also in vegetables such as artichokes, spinach and squash.

Probiotics – are live microorganisms that when administered in adequate amounts confer a health benefit on the host. Probiotics are commonly consumed as part of fermented foods with specially added active live cultures, such as in yogurt, soy yogurt, or as dietary supplements. Studies have shown that healthy stomach bacteria found in probiotics can help reduce inflammation and help lose weight. If you are getting your probiotics in yogurt be sure to avoid those high in sugar.

Protein (Powders or Shakes) – these are used in meal replacement shakes; protein is one of the main building blocks for muscle and bone. Additional protein is needed for those who exercise or more active. The primary protein used in shakes are whey and soy; whey is found in milk, it is fast absorbing but in your body for a shorter amount of time and is a good supplement after intense workouts. Soy protein is a plant based source of protein, easily digestible, known for its antioxidants and a good supplement for meal replacements.

Resveratrol – is part of plant compounds called polyphenols; these compounds are thought to have antioxidant properties, protecting the body against the kind of damage linked to increased risk for conditions such as cancer and heart disease. Resveratrol is found in the skin of red grapes, but other sources include peanuts and berries.

SAM-e – also known as S-adenosylmethionine, is a synthetic form of a compound formed naturally in the body from essential amino acids that are an energy-producing compound found in all cells in the body. It is used for depression, osteoarthritis, liver health and for PMS in women among other ailments.

Selenium – is mineral absorbed into the body through water and food such as fish, poultry and wheat. It is taken to help with under-active thyroid, high cholesterol and heart health. There are other ailments and diseases selenium is thought to aid but more research is needed.

Turmeric (Curcumin) – is a plant used as a spice, it has a warm and bitter flavor and is the main spice in curry. It is also believed to have medicinal purpose used for arthritis, upset stomach, osteoarthritis and inflammation; there are other medical issues such as cancer it is used for but more evidence is needed.

Vitamin A – is a vitamin that can be found in many fruits, vegetables, eggs, whole milk, butter, fortified margarine, meat, and oily saltwater fish or taken as a vitamin supplement. It is beneficial for the eyes, bones, teeth and of course skin; it also strengthens immunity.

Vitamin B12 – is commonly found in foods, such as fish, shellfish, meat, eggs, and dairy products. It is used to treat fatigue, heart disease, high cholesterol and to improve memory.

Vitamin C – The benefits of vitamin C include protection against immune system deficiencies, cardiovascular disease, prenatal health problems, eye disease, and can help with wrinkles. Sources include fresh fruits and vegetables but especially citrus fruits. It is beneficial to the immune system and infections and helps to increase the absorption of iron among other benefits. Too little vitamin C in the blood stream has been found to correlate with increased body fat and waist measurements.

Vitamin D – this vitamin can be found in foods such as fish, dairy, juices but most vitamin D is obtained through exposure to the sun. It aids with bone weakness and boosting the immune system. Results from several studies suggest that the addition of vitamin D to a reduced-calorie diet will lead to better weight loss.

Vitamin E – is found in many foods including eggs, fruits, vegetables, meat and poultry; it is beneficial to many body functions and is an antioxidant which helps to slow down processes that damage cells. It is found in enough foods that it's rare to be deficient in and although it is good for overall health there is nothing that shows it aids in weight loss.

Vitamin K – is essential for helping the blood clot after an injury or cut and for overall health especially for bones and heart health. Excellent sources of vitamin K are leafy green vegetables and it is also found in milk, oats and meat. Again, there are no links to weight loss.

Zinc – is used for boosting the immune system and is beneficial for many diseases and skin conditions. It is found in meats, seafood, dairy, legumes and whole grain. Zinc does not aid specifically in weight loss but is an essential vitamin for diet, metabolism and health.

These vitamins are typically absorbed in the body by foods we eat daily as long as you are following a healthy and balanced diet.

About the Author:

Like most women I can be a little obsessed with my weight and diet; but this is the only life I have and want to make it the best I can...I want to look good and I want to feel good. I'm also a little obsessed with being healthy and active when I reach my golden years which means taking care of myself now.

But I also love food, so I understand that there has to be a balance...the key word is "moderation". I find joy in living healthy without feeling deprived.

Working in the corporate world for years I understand how difficult it can be to eat healthy and find time for exercise. I also felt most books out there written by people whose full time job is fitness and nutrition didn't understand that issue or address it. Which is why I want to reach out to the typical working woman (and man) and together we can fight the diet struggle.

Linny Harris

www.DietStruggle.com

www.ingramcontent.com/pod-product-compliance
Lightning Source LLC
Chambersburg PA
CBHW060335290526
45793CB00003B/630